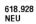

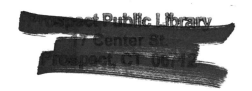

"I'm, Like, **SO** Fat!"

"I'm, Like, SO Fat!"

Helping Your Teen Make Healthy Choices about Eating and Exercise in a Weight-Obsessed World

Dianne Neumark-Sztainer, PhD

THE GUILFORD PRESS
New York   London

© 2005 Dianne Neumark-Sztainer
Published by The Guilford Press
A Division of Guilford Publications, Inc.
72 Spring Street, New York, NY 10012
www.guilford.com

The information in this volume is not intended as a substitute for consultation with health care professionals. Each individual's health concerns should be evaluated by a qualified professional.

Printed in the United States of America

This book is printed on acid-free paper.

Last digit is print number: 9   8   7   6   5   4   3   2   1

Library of Congress Cataloging-in-Publication Data

Neumark-Sztainer, Dianne.
    I'm, like, SO fat!: helping your teen make healthy choices about eating and exercise in a weight-obsessed world / Dianne Neumark-Sztainer.
        p.   cm.
    Includes bibliographical references and index.
    ISBN 1-57230-980-6 (pbk.) — ISBN 1-59385-167-7 (hardcover)
    1. Eating disorders in adolescence.   2. Teenagers—Health and hygiene.   3. Physical fitness for youth.   4. Physical fitness for children.   I. Title.
    RJ506.E18N48 2005
    618.92′8526—dc22
                                                            2004025953

This book is dedicated to the teens in my life who enrich it with their questions, thoughtfulness, challenges, love, and laughter: Shahar (soon to enter young adolescence), Maya (a middle adolescent), Tal (a late adolescent), and Lior (just finishing up adolescence and moving into young adulthood). May you grow up in a world in which a person's actions matter more than a person's appearance, and may your actions make this world a better place to live in.

Contents

**"How can we make a difference at home . . .
and away?"**

"What can we do when problems come up?"

Acknowledgments

*T*he process of writing this book had a number of parallels to the process of parenting teens. There was a lot of preparatory work to be done before even beginning, and I needed a lot of support along the way. As with parenting teens, things were easier and came out better because I had partners in the process. From the depths of my heart, I want to acknowledge all of those who contributed to the research that served as the basis for this book and led to its creation, and to those who supported the writing of this book once it became a reality.

Many thanks to all of my research partners, and especially to my friend and colleague Dr. Mary Story, who has been a part of much of the research that forms the basis of this book. Thanks to all of the Project EAT staff, especially Peter Hannan, Dr. Cheryl Perry, Dr. Marla Eisenberg, and Dr. Melanie Wall. Thanks also to Nicole Hanson, Jess Haines, and Annabel Kornblum for your many contributions.

Throughout the course of writing this book, I had the opportunity to travel to different countries and different places within the United States to meet with my eating disorder prevention colleagues. Thanks to all of you for your ideas and support with special thanks to Dr. Michael Levine, Dr. Niva Piran, Dr. Linda Smolak, Dr. Susan Paxton, and Dr. Eleanor Wertheim. Although our colleague Dr. Lori Irving died before this book got started, her enthusiasm for advocacy for young people and collaboration across the fields of eating disorder and obesity prevention were an impetus for pulling many of the ideas in this book together.

x   I am so grateful to the staff at The Guilford Press for your enthusiasm for this project and your help in getting it into the readers' hands in its current format. It has been an honor to work with you. Thanks particularly to Kitty Moore, Executive Editor, for your initial excitement about this book and making it happen. I want to offer a very special thanks to Christine Benton, my Developmental Editor, for all of your hard work. You have been a true partner every step of the way. You spiced up the pages and made the process truly fun. I look forward to our next project.

Along the way, many of my friends who are also parenting teens talked with me about their struggles to help their children develop healthy eating and exercise patterns *and* feel good about their bodies. Thank you for your stories . . . and more importantly for your friendship.

I can't imagine parenting my teens, or writing this book, without my husband, Hector Sztainer, who is always there for me. Thanks for your help with intangible items, such as your love for me, and more tangible support, such as driving kids, grocery shopping, and cooking family meals.

Finally, thanks to all of the teens that provided the ideas and the solutions that are presented throughout this book. Thank you for filling out surveys and participating in interviews. A special thanks to my own children, Lior, Tal, Maya, and Shahar, and your wonderful friends for answering all of my questions along the way. I hope you think the final result was worth it.

Introduction

"*I*'m, like, SO fat . . . why can't I look like Heather?"

"Ewwww, I can't eat THAT. Look at all that GREASE. . . . Wanna go get a Frappuccino?"

"I'm being really good today: I haven't eaten a single calorie."

"No, I'm not eating dinner, Dad; gotta make weight. I'll be at the gym, probably till you're in bed."

Sound familiar? Even fleeting encounters with teenagers today will tell you volumes about the pressures they're up against: "Supersize it" . . . but downsize yourself. "Just do it" . . . or just stay home watching reality TV and IM-ing your friends. Hang out at the mall with the other kids, where you'll feel worse and worse about not fitting into those size 1 designer jeans, until you finally console yourself with a fat-laden liquid dessert masquerading as coffee.

Our society is full of pressures that promote obesity but reward thinness. We're surrounded by high-calorie, low-nutrient food. Portion sizes have grown dramatically. Technological advances make it easy to get through the day without breaking a sweat. And I don't know what it's like where you live, but in my neighborhood kids aren't out playing tag and hide-and-seek like we used to do. Yet we're all supposed to stay thin and muscular.

No wonder our teenagers are confused—at best—and dissatisfied with the way they look. At worst they are suffering health-damaging excess weight, life-threatening eating disorders, or psychological pain that sends negative ripples through all aspects of their lives. We're seeing a continuing increase in eating- and weight-related problems ranging from obesity to body dissatisfaction, erratic eating patterns, binge eating, too much or too little physical activity, unhealthy weight control behaviors, and eating disorders.

Parents are at their wits' end. You're probably hearing lots of advice for preventing obesity and eating disorders in your sons and daughters, much of it likely conflicting, in part because it generally comes from separate fields of science. This leaves you without a clue about how to protect your child from the health hazards of obesity without inadvertently planting the seeds of an unhealthy weight obsession. You may wonder what to say to your kids to help them be more accepting of their bodies regardless of size or shape, while still encouraging healthy food choices and a physically active lifestyle. You want your daughter to rejoice in the changes occurring in her body as she enters adolescence, not cringe when she looks in the mirror or compares herself to the latest rock starlet. You want your 18-year-old son to make healthy food and exercise choices on his own when he moves to a college dorm or apartment. You want your kids to listen to what reliable sources have to say about nutrition and activity and health, not to what they hear from uninformed peers or commercial enterprises with a profit-making agenda to push. And you want to accomplish this without being an overbearing, overprotective, overcontrolling parent, insensitive to your teens' needs to become independent.

I want the same things. As the mother of four children at different stages of adolescence, I struggle with the same issues—how to raise my kids to feel good about their bodies, take care of their health, and avoid becoming overweight without yielding to extreme weight control measures. Fortunately, I've had the opportunity to explore these issues with many other teenagers and their parents over the past 20 years. I started off doing this within clinical settings, where I worked as a dietitian with teenagers and adults who were interested in weight management, struggling with eating disorders, or just wanting to improve their eating and physical activity behaviors. I am currently exploring issues related to parent–teen relations, family meal patterns, teen eating and physical activity behaviors, body image, dieting, steroid use, eating disorders, and obesity, as a researcher and professor in the School of Public Health at the University of Minnesota.

My colleagues, students, and I have been involved with various types of studies to address our research questions more fully and from different angles. We've conducted *qualitative* research, in which we interviewed teens to find out what they think about key issues such as factors that influence their food choices, family meals, what it feels like to grow up overweight in a thin-oriented society, and how their parents can help them adopt healthier behaviors and feel good about themselves. Throughout this book, reference will be made to the words of wisdom that the teens who participated in these studies shared with us.

We've also conducted *epidemiological* research, in which we surveyed large numbers of teens from diverse backgrounds to get a better picture of the major issues facing teens and their families today. The study that will be referred to most often in this book is Project EAT (Eating Among Teens), since it was designed specifically to learn more about eating patterns, physical activity, dieting behaviors, and weight concerns among teenagers. Project EAT is one of the largest and most comprehensive research studies to examine factors associated with eating patterns and weight-related issues in adolescents. In this study, 4,746 adolescents completed surveys and had their height and weight measured. In addition, we interviewed 900 of their parents by phone. One of my reasons for writing this book was to share the Project EAT findings with parents of teens.*

Based on what we learned from teens in qualitative research and epidemiological studies, we've developed interventions to address their concerns and conducted *intervention* research to see if these approaches are acceptable to teens and effective in bringing about change. We've developed and evaluated programs such as Very Important Kids for elementary school girls and boys, Free to Be Me for preteen Girl Scouts, The Weigh to Eat for high school girls and boys, and New Moves for high school girls. Each of these programs has taken a slightly different approach to preventing weight-related problems by promoting self-esteem, preventing teasing, enhancing media literacy skills, encouraging healthy eating, and making physical activity fun for teens of different shapes and sizes. Lessons learned from these and other studies, and ideas that can be used within homes and schools, are described in this book.

The beauty of this process is that it's cyclical. Each study provides answers but also raises more questions, which then lead to another research study. My experiences as a parent of teens have also led to new research questions, and, in turn, my research has informed my parenting. Through this

---

*If you are interested in learning more about Project EAT, see our website at *www.epi.umn. edu/research/eat*.

book, I hope our research will inform your parenting too. Finally, I hope that your experiences with using some of the ideas included here will enhance our body of knowledge and raise further questions to be addressed.

In our research we heard things from teens that they might not easily share with their own parents, which may make it possible for you to help your teens more effectively. There are no simple recipes for raising children, and I'm not going to try to sell you on "an easy five-step plan to success." Body image, self-esteem, eating patterns, body shape and size, physical activity behaviors—these are complex issues, and solutions will differ for different individuals and families. Yet I believe that given the knowledge we have gained, you'll be able to apply it in a manner that *makes the most sense for your family*.

So, this book is based on a substantial body of research done with teens and their families. My motivation for writing it was to synthesize the research findings and get them to the people who care about them most—you, the parents of teens and teens-to-be. Too often, research findings sit on the shelves of academics and are not made readily available to parents. I know how thirsty parents are for good, sound information to guide their actions. This book provides an integration of the findings from my own studies and many others going on in the field. I've made my best efforts to present the data clearly and to offer practical suggestions based on what we discovered. My hope is that as a result of your reading this book the teens in your life, and teens everywhere, will . . .

- accept and for the most part rejoice in their bodies and the changes occurring during adolescence;
- nurture and care for their bodies by staying involved in physical activities that they enjoy, eating healthy food, and avoiding unhealthy weight control and disordered eating behaviors;
- maintain a body weight that is healthy *for them* through healthy activity and eating, but also appreciate that different body shapes and sizes can be both healthy and beautiful;
- recognize that weightism is unacceptable and refuse to be the victims, supporters, or perpetrators of weight stigmatization; and
- work toward making our environment more conducive to healthy physical activity and eating behaviors *and* more accepting of diverse body shapes and sizes.

This book is divided into five sections. In the first two, I lay the foundation for the rest of the book by explaining what I mean by weight-related problems and delving into all the factors that contribute to them in our teenagers, ranging from our own issues with weight and body image to the influence of peers and media, the role of physical activity, the myths about dieting, and the realities of adolescent development. At the end of the second section, I offer some guidelines for working toward the goal we all want to achieve: preventing both obesity *and* eating disorders in our teens.

The third and fourth sections get into the specifics that we all have to deal with in our daily home life. The perennial questions about what and how much kids should eat are addressed in the third section (Chapters 8–10), which offer science-based answers to questions such as: What are some alternatives to dieting? How do you instill a solid understanding of and respect for nutrition in kids who might find the subject about as fascinating as the migration habits of the blue-breasted nuthatch? Is it helpful or harmful to talk to your teens about portion control and calories? And what do you need to consider if they announce they're becoming vegetarians? In the fourth section (Chapters 11–13) we'll look at how you get there once you've decided what a healthy diet means for your teens and your family—what role family meals should play and how you can make them happen in our peripatetic world, how you can make the best of eating out, and, finally, how to talk to your testy, sensitive teens when any of a wide variety of very complicated, very typical problems surrounding eating, weight, and body image arise.

The last section of the book is for those of you who have an overweight teenager or a teenager who has (or who you suspect may have) an eating disorder. There's a lot you can do to help, all of it based on the principles and data presented earlier in the book.

In this book, I've tried to distill everything I've learned in my research, from thousands of open and honest teens and their parents, and from my own trial-and-error parenting. Reading this book and incorporating its ideas can help you raise teenagers who like their bodies and treat them with respect, who relish good food and take joy in movement, who will protect themselves from the side effects of excess weight but won't sweat a few extra pounds, a week away from the gym, or the changes that come naturally as they mature.

You can make a big difference. I hope this book will show you how.

"I'm, Like, **SO** Fat!"

"What are we up against ... and how did we get here, anyway?"

1

If It's Not One Thing, It's Another

Dealing with a Spectrum of Weight-Related Problems

Sarah is 12 and going through puberty. Like many girls her age, she's spending more and more time in front of the mirror. While she's there, she talks to herself—"I look *SO* fat"—and makes faces, pinching the flesh on her newly rounded hips.

David just got his driver's license, and now a few times a week dinner is a burger with fries or a Super Grande "Works" Burrito instead of a home-cooked meal with his family.

Home for a visit after her first semester at college, Amanda has lost 15 pounds. The food at school is "horrendously disgusting," she protests while pushing her dad's specialty pasta primavera around on her plate. The next morning her parents awake with a start when they hear the front door slam at five o'clock and look out the window to see their customarily late-rising daughter jogging down the street.

When Joe comes home from middle school, the first thing he does is tell his mother how much he hates his school because the kids are so mean about his weight. The second thing he does is grab some chips and soda pop and sit down in front of the TV.

Maybe you know some of these kids. Possibly you've got one like them living in your house. If you do, you probably have the same worries their parents have. Is Sarah just going through a phase of negativity about her body? Will David's health start to suffer if he keeps substituting burgers and fries for balanced dinners? Why is Amanda behaving so differently—is something wrong? And can Joe's mom help him accept himself and reject the cruelty of teasing while also encouraging him to change habits that contribute to overweight? Can she do so without sounding like she's taking sides with the kids who demean her son?

Joe's mother is facing the dilemma we're all up against today: It's hard enough to find answers to the questions that come up about weight, food, exercise, body shape, and all the physical, mental, and emotional health factors connected to these topics. But even when we do have some of the answers, how do we *talk* to our kids in a positive, productive way? My goal in this book is to help you with both.

Most teenagers experience some type of eating-, activity-, or weight-related problem as they transition from childhood to adulthood. For some teens these problems are mild; for others they can be quite extreme. Often the progression of a problem and its final outcome depend on its early identification and appropriate intervention. That's why it's so important to seek answers to your questions and then act on them.

The trouble is, it's all so complicated. Joe's mother knows it's right to make her son feel good about himself and to instill in him zero tolerance for taunting people about their appearance. What mother wouldn't? She also knows her son would probably lose some weight if he did something active after school rather than watching TV and ate snacks composed of something other than junk food. But if she tries to deliver these messages simultaneously, she's afraid that one message might cancel out the other. So how *does* she handle it?

The parents of the other kids face similar challenges. Sarah's parents want to assure her that her body is normal and that she can take pride and enjoyment in maturing. But they also want her to know that she's made up of a lot more than flesh and bones and that she has many other strengths. How can they make her feel good about her body without making it seem disproportionately important in a world that tells her it is? And how do they know whether she's just going through a phase that will pass as it should if they *don't* say anything?

Amanda's parents have more pressing concerns: Their daughter has lost a lot of weight and seems determined to lose more. Is she developing an eating disorder? What will happen to her once she goes back to school and is away from their watchful eyes? What can they do right now to protect Amanda from unhealthy weight loss? What *shouldn't* they do—to ensure that the lines of communication stay open?

David's parents want to allow him the freedom he's earned, but they don't want it to undo all the good work they've done to instill healthy eating habits over the previous 16 years. And they miss having him at the dinner table, where they can find out about what he's been up to all day. They're now realizing what they've always taken for granted—that family meals are not just about food.

If issues like these aren't complicated enough, there are the mixed messages that we're barraged with: Pick up a super-duper-sized, fat-laden quick-fix lunch at the drive-through every day, but make sure you can fit into that size-2 swimsuit. Play a sport, get buff, join a health club, no excuses—unless, of course, you're too busy trying to beat the newest videogame or you just have to catch the latest reality show episode. Go ahead and treat yourself to dinner at the new gourmet Italian place, but when they plunk a plate mounded with pasta in front of you, try not to eat more than a third of it. As adults we all fall prey to such pressures, and it's easy to pass on our confusion and ambivalence to our kids. Imagine how hard it is for teenagers to sort out everything they see and hear about food, exercise, and body image. Many of them can't, with the result that the prevalence of weight-related problems among our sons and daughters has never been higher, and their consequences have never been as serious:

- The prevalence of obesity in teenagers has tripled over the past 20 years. Currently 15% of teenage girls and boys are overweight.
- An additional 15–20% of teenage girls and boys are at risk of becoming overweight.
- Over one-half of teenage girls and nearly one-third of teenage boys use unhealthy weight control behaviors such as skipping meals, fasting, smoking cigarettes, vomiting, and taking laxatives.
- Dieting has been found to lead to weight gain, and not to weight loss, in teenagers.
- Girls who diet frequently are 12 times as likely to binge eat as girls who don't diet, and boys who diet frequently are at a 7 times greater risk for binge eating.
- One-half of teenage girls and one-fourth of teenage boys are dissatisfied with their bodies.

- Approximately 1 out of 200 adolescent girls and young women develop anorexia nervosa.
- The prevalence of bulimia nervosa is 1–3% among adolescent girls and young women. Thus, out of 100 females, 1–3 will develop bulimia nervosa.
- Although eating disorders are more common among girls than boys, a significant number of teenage boys develop serious eating disorders, and many more engage in harmful weight-loss or muscle-gain behaviors.

Undoubtedly, you've already heard some of these statistics. You can hardly help it when it seems impossible to open a magazine or newspaper or watch television without reading or hearing about weight-related problems: "The new obesity epidemic!" "Lose five pounds in one week without breaking a sweat!" "Award-winning pop artist admits she has an eating disorder!" When I see the cover of a major magazine such as *Newsweek* or *Time* focusing on the "obesity epidemic," I have mixed feelings. As someone who works in the field, I'm pleased that weight-related problems are getting the attention they deserve. Unless we take problems such as the increasing prevalence of obesity among children seriously, they will continue. But I also get concerned about how vulnerable individuals may react when the alarm is sounded. I get particularly worried about teenagers, who may already have excessive concerns about their weight and appearance. On one side of the tightrope that we're forced to walk today is the risk of obesity; on the other, the risk of eating disorders. How do we keep our balance?

I believe the only answer is to consider all the weight-related issues together.

Why We Need to View Weight-Related Problems as a Spectrum

Too often when we address eating-, activity-, and weight-related problems, we focus on only one issue. When I say "we," by the way, I mean my colleagues and I in scientific research, doctors treating patients, journalists, and parents— all of us. We may worry about preventing obesity without paying enough attention to promoting a positive body image or preventing eating disorders. Sometimes we dismiss mild problems, such as skipping meals, body dissatisfaction, or unhealthy dieting, as normal for teens and wait until such problems become more severe to intervene. As the kids introduced at the beginning of this chapter illustrate, however, we aren't one-dimensional, and neither are our weight-related problems. Therefore, over the years I've become more and more convinced that we need to:

1. *Pay attention to the different types of weight-related problems.* In trying to get our kids to make healthier food choices, we don't want our efforts to lead to an obsession with counting fat grams or calories. In trying to prevent eating disorders in our teens, we cannot ignore the dangers associated with being overweight.
2. *Be alert to mild shades of weight-related problems.* We can't afford to wait until our teens develop eating disorders to intervene; we need to step in much earlier. When they say things like "I feel so fat" or "I'm starting a diet tomorrow," we need to have a constructive response. We need to pay attention to the number of family meals they have missed recently or the disappearance of food from the kitchen.

The spectrum of weight-related problems includes five dimensions, ranging from healthy to problematic (as illustrated from left to right):

1. Weight control practices, from healthy eating to clinical eating disorders.
2. Physical activity, from moderate to either excessive or absent.
3. Body image, from satisfied to very dissatisfied.
4. Eating behaviors, from regular eating practices to binge eating.
5. Weight status, from healthy to severely underweight or overweight.

These five dimensions are interrelated and, in fact, can be tightly intertwined in any one person. This means that when you see one problem in your child, other problems may lie below the surface or may appear in the future. Sixteen-year-old Karen is overweight, so she begins to experiment with fad diets. She says she hates what she sees in the mirror and absolutely has to lose weight before the prom. Seeing how unhappy she is, and knowing the health risks that come with obesity, Karen's mother naturally wants to help her move toward a healthier weight. But that will involve more than putting balanced meals and reasonable portions on the table to steer her daughter away from a crash diet. She'll also need to help Karen develop a positive body image, override the influence of peers and advertisers who tell her that she can lose 30 pounds in 30 days, help her find physical activities that appeal to her, and help

	Healthy →	→	→	Problematic
Weight control practices:	Healthy eating	Dieting	Unhealthy weight control behaviors	Anorexia or bulimia nervosa
Physical activity behaviors:	Moderate physical activity	Minimal or excessive activity	Lack of, or obsessive, physical activity	"Anorexia athletica"
Body image:	Body acceptance	Mild body dissatisfaction	Moderate body dissatisfaction	Severe body dissatisfaction
Eating behaviors:	Regular eating patterns	Erratic eating behaviors	Binge eating	Binge eating disorder
Weight status:	Healthy body weight	Mildly overweight or underweight	Overweight or underweight	Severe overweight or underweight
	Healthy →	→	→	**Problematic**

The spectrum of eating-, activity-, and weight-related concerns.

her avoid binge eating. Unless Karen and her parents look at all the dimensions on the spectrum, they won't have much success in solving the surface problem and may inadvertently trigger additional problems.

The use of the spectrum also makes it easy to address budding problems early, when they are easier to solve. Too often parents and doctors get stuck in the dichotomy of "normal" versus "abnormal." When we can say, "No, this teenager doesn't have a serious problem," we absolve ourselves of the need to do anything about that gut feeling that something is not quite right—until we are forced to say, "Yes, now there is a serious problem." Then we intervene. Sarah, described in the first scenario at the beginning of this chapter, has normal developmental concerns about the changes going on in her body. Her parents can help prevent these concerns from blossoming into more serious problems in a slew of different ways. They can talk to Sarah about the normal changes that occur during adolescence. They can make an active effort to be positive role models. They can stay aware of the messages their daughter is getting from the media and advocate for positive, healthy advertising and marketing. And they can explore what Sarah really means when she says she feels fat. If they think about weight-related problems as falling along a continuum, from mild to severe, Sarah's parents won't wait until their daughter is in real trouble to take these and other kinds of actions.

OBESITY AND EATING DISORDERS: NOT SO FAR APART AFTER ALL

Traditionally, obesity and eating disorders have been viewed as distinct conditions. Yet research is beginning to reveal that they can be intertwined. In our own research, we found that overweight teenagers are at high risk of using unhealthy weight control behaviors and engaging in binge eating behaviors. In addition, individuals can cross over from one condition to another over time. Dr. Christopher Fairburn and his colleagues found that adult women with bulimia nervosa and women with binge eating disorder were more likely to have been overweight during childhood than comparison groups. They also found that exposure to weight-related comments and teasing increased the women's risk for the later onset of a clinical eating disorder. Research findings, clinical impressions, and personal experiences strongly suggest that excessive social pressure on overweight individuals to be thin can increase their risk for unhealthy weight control behaviors and even clinical eating disorders. Consequently, we can no longer think in terms of just one problem; rather, we need to pay attention to the broad spectrum of eating-, activity-, and weight-related problems.

	Teenage girls	Teenage boys
Unhealthy weight control behaviors (for example, skipping meals, eating very little, fasting, or smoking for weight loss)	57%	33%
Dieting behaviors	55%	26%
Body dissatisfaction	46%	26%
Extreme weight control behaviors (for example, vomiting, use of laxatives, diet pills)	12%	5%
Binge eating behaviors	17%	8%
Obesity	15%	15%
Moderately overweight/at risk for overweight	15–20%	15–20%
Binge eating disorder	3–5%	1–3%
Bulimia nervosa	1–3%	<1%
Anorexia nervosa	0.5%	<0.2%

These data are from Project EAT and other large studies on teenagers and young adults.

Maybe the figures in the table come as a surprise to you. Maybe they just confirm what you've suspected all along about the magnitude of weight-related problems among our teens. To protect our sons and daughters, however, we have to know where the dangers lie. Let's take a closer look at each dimension and the hazards lurking at the extreme ends of each.

I. Weight Control Practices: Reasonable or Irrational?

How many people do you know who have never dieted? In our society, dieting is so common as to seem normal. But that doesn't mean it's harmless, particularly in children and teens. For some teens, the feelings of hunger and deprivation that often accompany dieting lead to binge eating and, somewhat ironically, to weight gain. Research has also shown that all too often simple dieting can turn into unhealthy dieting, and in some teens can be the first step toward a more problematic eating disorder. How to prevent dieting from causing problems for your teen is discussed throughout this book, particularly in Chapter 6. The key features of some of the more severe eating disorders are described here.

ANOREXIA NERVOSA: NOT JUST TOO MUCH DIETING, BUT THAT CAN BE WHERE IT BEGINS

Anorexia nervosa is perhaps the most severe condition included on the spectrum of weight-related disorders. It's a very serious illness, requiring long-term treatment with a health care team that specializes in eating disorders. If you suspect your child may be developing this problem, it's essential that you contact a professional immediately. Also read Chapter 15.

Characteristics of anorexia nervosa include self-starvation and a strong fear of being fat. Some of the symptoms include weight loss, severe body image disturbances, dry skin, intolerance to cold, fatigue, constipation, and irregular menstrual cycles, although not all of these may appear. Teens may develop unusual eating habits, such as limiting the types of foods they are willing to eat, avoiding family meals, pushing food around on the plate, cutting food into small pieces, and weighing or portioning food. They may engage in intense and compulsive physical activity as another weight control strategy.

Teens often begin the process by dieting for weight control purposes, but as dieting behaviors lead to weight loss, feelings of control, and compliments from others about weight loss, anorexia nervosa can develop in vulnerable individuals. Once it does develop, anorexia nervosa seems to take on a life of its own as the need for control over eating, activity, and other behaviors becomes extreme and somewhat obsessive. Consider the scenario, at the beginning of this chapter, about Amanda, who has just returned from college and appears to be displaying anorexic behaviors. Although her parents are concerned, Amanda may be getting compliments from others about her weight loss. These compliments can reinforce her unhealthy behaviors. I have seen this happen many times, and it is very disturbing to concerned family members who are aware of the underlying problems that others may not be seeing and are inadvertently reinforcing. Imagine how 13-year-old Linda's parents felt when she returned from long-term inpatient hospital treatment for anorexia nervosa and her neighbors, remembering how overweight Linda had been when younger, complimented her on how good she looked at her lower weight! About nine out of ten individuals with anorexia nervosa are female.

This doesn't mean you should ignore the signs of anorexia nervosa in your son, however. Because of its relative rarity in males, it is possible for health care providers, educators, and parents to overlook those signs in boys, which means the condition may be recognized only in its later stages, when treatment may be more challenging.

Unfortunately, denial of anorexia nervosa by a teenager and family members is common. This is understandable, since it's extremely difficult for parents to accept the fact that their child is starving him- or herself. One of the first things a mother does after giving birth is to feed her infant; this is the basis for the beginning of a relationship. Not having food to give to one's child, or having a child who refuses to eat in the midst of plenty, is one of the toughest things a parent will ever face. But if a teacher or friend raises concerns about your teen, resist any knee-jerk denial, listen to what you're being told, and take a close look at your child.

BULIMIA NERVOSA:
YOU MAY NEED TO LOOK HARDER TO FIND IT

In bulimia nervosa the affected person cycles between eating large amounts of food and trying to get rid of the food consumed through self-induced vomiting, laxative use, strict dieting, fasting, or excessive exercising. Those with bulimia nervosa often experience feelings of failure and lack of control because of bingeing behaviors, which interfere with weight loss. School performance, relationships, and self-esteem can suffer dramatically. Teens with limited resources may steal money to buy food for their binges. They can end up with dental problems, throat irritations, stomach cramps, heartburn, and more severe electrolyte imbalances and cardiac irregularities. Sometimes a dentist will be the first to suspect the illness, because vomiting can lead to enamel erosion and cavities.

As with anorexia nervosa, approximately nine out of ten cases of bulimia nervosa are found in females, but males do develop bulimia nervosa, so it's important to be aware of any suspicious behaviors in adolescent boys and young men. Bulimia nervosa also tends to be more common among college-age adolescents than among middle school or high school students.

Be aware that those who have bulimia nervosa often try to hide their behaviors because of their fear of being discovered, embarrassment, and shame. In contrast to those with anorexia nervosa, who often exhibit severe weight loss, individuals with bulimia nervosa tend to maintain their weight within a 5- to 10-pound range or may show large weight fluctuations due to alternating bingeing and purging behaviors. This can make it harder to notice bulimia nervosa by just looking at your son or daughter. Many years ago, Dina, who was in a weight control group that I ran, told me how she would consume several whole loaves of bread at a time. Dina hid her behaviors from other family members and would sometimes go into a closet to eat. At the time, I did not know much about eating disorders, and I found it hard to believe that she ate so much since she had a lean body. I still regret not fully understanding her condition and giving her the help she was asking for. If missing food and/ or money leads you to suspect that your teen is engaging in bulimic behaviors, don't ignore your suspicions. Again, remember that the power of denial can be strong, and do your best to overcome your natural tendency to deny that a problem exists. Excellent treatment options are available for bulimia nervosa, and recovery rates are high.

2. Physical Activity: Most of Us Need to Move More . . . But Too Much Is Also a Problem

The major problem facing all of us within a world of cars, remote control, and computers is a lack of physical activity. I can get through my day without much movement unless I make an effort to go for a walk, ride my bike, or lift some weights. Do you have a teen who spends too much time in front of a screen? We'll come back to some strategies for helping that child to get a bit more active in Chapter 5.

Although most teens are not doing enough in the way of physical activity, some are doing too much. *Anorexia athletica* is not recognized as a formal eating disorder, but the term has gained increasing use because of the recognition that excessive and compulsive physical activity can be harmful. Since it has not been recognized as a formal eating disorder, criteria for defining this condition have not been established and no estimates of its prevalence have been made; thus, at first I hesitated to include it in this discussion. However, I think it is important to consider here. Too often physical activity is presented as the be-all and end-all to solving obesity and eating disorders. The fact that any excess can be a problem illustrates the importance of viewing all of these dimensions in our spectrum as falling along a continuum.

What should you watch for here? I'd be concerned about teens who appear to engage in excessive exercise beyond the requirement for good health, steal time to exercise whenever feasible, have lost a sense of enjoyment in being physically active, and define their self-worth in terms of their level of phys-

A Spectrum of Weight-Related Problems

ical activity. It may be that a teen has anorexia nervosa and is using exercise as the main route to weight loss. I remember seeing an excellent video in which a young woman realizes that she has a problem when she is about to complete a marathon and is already thinking about going to the gym. Teens engaging in excessive physical activity for weight control purposes definitely need to be evaluated for an eating or exercise disorder.

3. Body Image: Dissatisfaction Is a Problem

Isn't body dissatisfaction part of being a teen? No, it doesn't have to be. Does it really matter? Yes, it does. In the Project EAT study, described in the Introduction to this book, 46% of teenage girls and 26% of boys expressed dissatisfaction with their bodies. This will come as no surprise to the parents of a teenager. But it's like dieting: Just because it's prevalent doesn't mean it's benign. Research has shown that body dissatisfaction is closely linked to self-esteem in adolescents, more so than in adults. This isn't surprising either, but we sometimes lose sight of how significant it is. A key task of adolescence is to develop one's self-concept and sense of identity; body dissatisfaction can definitely interfere with that milestone of development. Body dissatisfaction can also lead to depression in teenagers and is probably the strongest risk factor for the use of unhealthy weight control behaviors. If we take these links seriously, it's clear that body dissatisfaction should *not* be viewed as a normal and acceptable component of adolescent development.

The teens who participated in our research studies were acutely aware of the far-reaching effects of a positive body image; they described how feeling good about your body instills a positive attitude, which attracts friends and gives you confidence, which helps you in your chosen career. On the flip side, severe body dissatisfaction can make it difficult for teenagers to accept compliments, describe themselves in positive terms, or even participate in activities that they might otherwise enjoy, such as dancing, swimming, or going to a party. If your child has a serious problem with body image, you might hear her constantly comparing herself negatively to peers, family members, and celebrities or models. She might begin to equate thinness with happiness and success, saying all of her problems would be solved and life would be different "if only" she were "skinnier" or had smaller hips or a narrower waist. When our research team interviewed larger-than-average teenagers, many of them expressed unforgiving disgust with their own images in the mirror. Some said they wished they could literally cut off the bulging parts of their bodies—a wish that recent television makeover shows seem to promise to fulfill. Ideally, overweight teens should recognize that their weight may be higher than is healthy for them and work toward making changes in their eating and physical activity behaviors, yet should still be able to appreciate their positive aspects and view themselves with respect. We'll be coming back to how to achieve this balance throughout this book.

Teens need to be reminded about their positive traits. We can comment on our teens' physical appearance: "Your haircut looks great." But we also need to comment on other characteristics to help our teens broaden their self-image: "I love the way you express yourself" or "You have such a generous way of relating to your friends." We often do this with our younger children, but we sometimes forget that our older children also care about what we think. As I wrote this, in fact, I realized that I hadn't been very diligent in this regard myself. So I've been inserting comments into my conversations with my four children such as, "You really seem to have gotten into your studies this semester," "I loved watching you play tennis today," "You have a real knack for understanding where people are coming from," or "You are so amazing at math." They're all true; I just need to remember to say them.

what you can do
IF THEY DON'T LIKE WHAT THEY SEE IN THE MIRROR, TELL THEM TO LOOK AGAIN TOMORROW

I have a friend whose pediatrician got her daughter on the right path with just a few wise words that my friend never forgot. When the daughter was 10 or 11, the doctor told her, "A lot's going to be happening to your body over the next six or seven years. Sometimes you're going to love your body, and sometimes you're going to hate it. Whenever you don't like it, just wait—it's going to change again." The warmth and we're-all-in-this-together sense with which the female doctor delivered this critical message may have been just as effective as her words. My friend could see the relief in her daughter's responding smile. And over the next few years, whenever her daughter said she couldn't stand the way she looked, my friend reminded her of what her doctor had told her. Every time, that memory brought the same relieved smile to her face. Why not try the same message with your own kids? It will go a long way toward establishing an identity that includes acceptance for the body and the many changes it will experience through life.

A Spectrum of Weight-Related Problems

4. Eating Behaviors: Erratic and Emotional Eating in Teens

Does your teenager eat when hungry and stop when full, eat regular meals, choose orange juice instead of soda pop, and sometimes eat a bit of dessert? If so, skip this section . . . your daughter or son is probably at the healthy end of the spectrum for eating behaviors. Eating as a response to physical hunger, on a fairly regular basis throughout the day, and according to the food pyramid (Chapter 8) is an important goal for all teens.

The reality, however, is that many teenagers overeat in response to a hard day, to deal with difficult emotions, or just when there is good food around (so, for that matter, do a lot of adults). Many adolescents also go for long periods without eating and then get so hungry that they consume large amounts of foods in an uncontrolled manner. All of us do this to some extent, but it can become problematic when it occurs on a regular basis and becomes a pattern, when large amounts of food are consumed, and when the "extra" eating is followed by feelings of guilt, remorse, disgust, or shame. If a teen overeats at Thanksgiving, I wouldn't give it another thought. I would, however, worry about a teen who has been eating full boxes of cookies, ice cream by the gallon, or large bags of potato chips, often enough that it is having a significant impact on your grocery bill. I would be concerned about a kid who gets down on himself for overeating and either talks about it ("I am so mad at myself for eating all that. I have no self-control") or shows other signs of remorse such as moodiness or social withdrawal. Since binge eating may be done secretly, I would also be concerned about the disappearance of food.

Binge eating disorder, shown at the far right on the spectrum for the eating behaviors dimension, is a condition characterized by frequently eating large amounts of food and feeling out of control during these eating episodes. *Frequently* is generally defined as "an average of at least two times a week for six months." Sometimes binge eating disorder may be referred to as compulsive overeating. People who binge are known to eat more rapidly than usual and continue even when uncomfortably full. They often feel guilty and depressed following the binge, which can lead to bingeing again, creating a cycle of binge eating. Binge eating is often done alone because of feelings of shame or embarrassment. Binge eating disorder differs from bulimia nervosa in that binges are not generally followed by purging or other compensatory behaviors, such as extreme dieting or excessive physical activity. Although individuals of all body weights can have binge eating disorder, it is more common among overweight individuals. Binge eating can lead to psychological and physical conditions, including depression, obesity, high cholesterol, diabetes, and heart disease. Among college students and adult populations, binge eating disorder is estimated to occur in about 5% of females and 3% of males. In younger teens who participated in Project EAT, the estimates were about 3% of females and 1% of males. Thus, gender differences are much smaller than those found for anorexia and bulimia nervosa.

Teens may engage in binge eating without having binge eating disorder. In Project EAT, 16% of average-weight teenage girls and 6% of average-weight teenage boys answered "yes" to the question "In the past year, have you ever eaten so much food in a short period of time that you would be embarrassed if others saw you (binge eating)?" Binge eating was more common in overweight teens than in average-weight teens; 21% of overweight adolescent girls and 12% of overweight adolescent boys reported binge eating.

Why are overweight individuals more likely to binge than others? Overweight teens report binge eating as a coping mechanism for dealing with stressful social situations, such as being teased about their weight or being excluded from friendship groups or sports teams, and with difficult emotions associated with high levels of body dissatisfaction. Ironically, this pattern just perpetuates a cycle in which the teenager gains more weight, continues to "feel so fat," and then just gives in to sitting in front of the TV and bingeing.

Obviously, it's important to work toward breaking this cycle, and there are various points in the chain of events that offer opportunities. An obvious one is the point at which the need for a coping mechanism arises. Parents can help their kids learn healthier coping mechanisms for dealing with difficult emotions and social situations by modeling and gently suggesting healthier alternatives such as listening to music, talking with friends, taking a hot bath, or going for a walk. As discussed in Chapter 6, avoiding restrictive dieting practices can make teens less vulnerable to binge eating in times of stress. Another point at which the cycle may be broken is before a particular stress is imposed on the teenager. Can we prevent teasing and make our adolescents feel accepted and loved regardless of their shape or size? There are a number of ways to encourage this attitude in friends and family provided throughout this book.

5. Weight Status:
The Challenges of Being Different

We need to pay more attention to the needs of overweight teens. As I discuss in Chapter 4, weight stigmatization is all too common in our society. All teens, but particularly overweight teens, are affected by it. The strong pressures on overweight youth to be thin increase their risk for unhealthy weight control behaviors, disordered eating behaviors, and eating disorders. In Project EAT, *nearly one-fifth (18%) of overweight girls and 6% of overweight boys reported that for weight control purposes they had made themselves vomit or taken laxatives, diuretics, or diet pills in the last year. Seventy-six percent of overweight girls and 55% of overweight boys reported unhealthy, although less extreme, weight control behaviors such as skipping meals, smoking, fasting, using food substitutes, and eating very little food.* These behaviors are not likely to be effective and may even lead to weight gain! Furthermore, they can be very harmful.

If you are the parent of an overweight teen, it's important to be aware of his or her increased risk for engaging in unhealthy weight control behaviors and experiencing the associated complications, including, but not limited to, the onset of an eating disorder. Some health care providers look for these behaviors only in very thin kids, and overweight teens may be overlooked. Parents are the gatekeepers to help for these teenagers.

A supportive home environment can greatly reduce the contribution of childhood obesity to the development of psychological problems and the use of unhealthy weight control behaviors. One teen we interviewed said her adult siblings encouraged her to try when she protested that she wanted to lose weight but couldn't, yet she emphasized that her family was "more concerned about me as a person than about my weight" and always provided support. Another teenager attributed her commitment to avoid purging behaviors for weight loss to a supportive family. It can be hard to parent a larger child within a society such as ours that places so much emphasis on thinness. Parents of larger children often find themselves in a bind about how to help . . . and not make things worse. Strategies for helping your overweight child with healthy weight management—without impairing your child's self-esteem, inadvertently prompting the use of extreme weight loss behaviors, or adding stress to your relationship—are discussed throughout this book, particularly in Chapter 14.

Eating-, Activity-, and Weight-Related Problems: Where Does My Child Fit In?

Take a few moments to fill out the following questionnaire that asks about your own child's attitudes and behaviors. If you have more than one child, complete the questionnaire separately for each child, or do it for the child who most concerns you. For ease of reading, some of the questions refer to girls and others to boys; all should be answered for your child, regardless of gender. Carefully considering the answers will better equip you to make decisions about how to move toward the healthy end of the spectrum.

WHERE IS YOUR CHILD ON THE SPECTRUM FOR EATING, ACTIVITY, AND WEIGHT-RELATED PROBLEMS?

			Circle one	
1. Does your teen experiment with different diets?	M	Yes	No
2. Does your child talk about looking forward to dance class, soccer practice, or any other sports?	H	Yes	No
3. Does your teen enjoy picking out new clothes and feel she knows what looks good on her?	H	Yes	No
4. Does your child eat regular meals?	H	Yes	No
5. Has your physician said anything negative about your child's weight status—that your child is underweight or overweight?	M	Yes	No
6. Does your teen play a sport, jog, attend a dance class, or follow an exercise program a few times a week for an hour or so each time?	H	Yes	No
7. Given the choice, would your teen usually choose to watch television over roller-blading, ice skating, or some other sport?	M	Yes	No
8. Do you have reason to believe, because of what you've heard from your teen or someone else, that your teen is being hurt by being teased about her body?	P	Yes	No
9. Does your child overeat whenever appealing food is around?	P	Yes	No
10. Does your child drop out of games or sports or other physical activity before the other kids because of tiring easily due to being overweight?	M	Yes	No
11. Does your teen eat a variety of foods, including fruits and vegetables, every day?	H	Yes	No
12. Does your teen spend his days running from activity to activity and spending his time in his bedroom doing jumping jacks or sit-ups?	P	Yes	No
13. If you asked your teen to describe himself, would he list all of his physical flaws before his strengths?	M	Yes	No *(cont.)*

From *"I'm, Like, SO Fat!"* by Dianne Neumark-Sztainer. Copyright 2005 by Dianne Neumark-Sztainer.

A Spectrum of Weight-Related Problems

14. Does your teen tend to eat a lot of foods that are low in nutrients and high in fats and sugars?	M	Yes	No
15. Does your teen's weight allow him to play the sports he likes and do as well as he would like?	H	Yes	No
16. Do you ever notice the smell of vomit in the bathroom after your teen has been there or find empty laxative packages in the garbage?	P	Yes	No
17. Does your teen seem distressed when she can't get to the health club that day or when she has to cut a practice short?	P	Yes	No
18. Does your teen explain not going to a dance, or not trying out for a team, as a result of being "fat" or "bad at sports"?	M	Yes	No
19. Does your child eat when hungry and stop eating when full?	H	Yes	No
20. Has your child's weight, in relation to his height, tended to be consistent over the years?	H	Yes	No
21. Does your teen talk about wanting to go on a diet?	M	Yes	No
22. Does your child like a variety of physical activities, including nonstructured activities such as walking and biking and structured activities like soccer team and dance class?	H	Yes	No
23. Has your teen suddenly started comparing his body negatively with everyone else's, to the point of refusing to go swimming, starting to wear nothing but baggy clothes, or giving up a sport?	P	Yes	No
24. Does your child tend to munch when nervous, sad, stressed, or angry?	P	Yes	No
25. Does your child seem too weak to keep up with the other kids because of being underweight?	P	Yes	No
26. Does your teen often engage in behaviors such as pushing food around the plate, cutting food into small pieces, or preparing food for others without eating it?	P	Yes	No
27. On average, does your child spend more than two hours a day watching television, playing video games, or doing nonschool activities on the computer?	M	Yes	No
28. If you asked your child to list five things she likes about herself, would she be able to do this?	H	Yes	No
29. Does your child skip meals on a regular basis?	M	Yes	No
30. Has your child recently had a large change in weight—either weight loss or weight gain?	P	Yes	No

SCORING THE QUIZ

What Is Your Teen's Overall Position on the Spectrum?

How many "yes" responses did you have for H questions? ____
How many "yes" responses did you have for M questions? ____
How many "yes" responses did you have for P questions? ____

The questionnaire contains 10 *H* questions, 10 *M* questions, and 10 *P* questions. A "perfect" score would include 10 "yes" responses for the *H* questions and zero "yes" responses for the *M* and *P* questions. Why? Because *H* indicates a healthy behavior, *M* a behavior that's moving toward problematic, and *P* a problematic behavior. Where does your child stand? Where is there room for improvement?

Where Is Your Teen in Regard to Specific Dimensions Shown on the Spectrum?

Now count the number of "yes" responses for questions marked with either an *M* or a *P* for each dimension. Do any of the dimensions appear to be problematic for your child? Even one "yes" response to a *P* question can indicate that there is a serious problem in that dimension.

Dimension on spectrum	Relevant questions	Number of "yes" responses
Weight control practices	1, 16, 21, 26	____
Physical activity behaviors	7, 12, 17, 27	____
Body image	8, 13, 18, 23	____
Eating regularity	9, 14, 24, 29	____
Weight status	5, 10, 25, 30	____

So, What Should You Do about What You've Learned?

- If your children are in the healthy range for most of these dimensions, your task will be to help them stay there as they go through adolescence. This book can help you prevent their progression toward the problematic end of the spectrum by keeping you apprised of the issues your kids are facing and helping you take some steps to stave off negative influences.

• If the questionnaire revealed that your son or daughter is moving toward the problematic in some dimension, this book will provide you with the skills to help your teen progress toward the healthier end of the spectrum. This may mean taking the same steps as for kids who are still in the healthy range but making a more concerted, targeted effort. It may also mean spending some time right now to find out more about the budding problem specifically or the whole spectrum of issues generally. You'll find tips for communicating in Chapters 7 and 13 that can be helpful if you have any hesitation about talking to your teen about these subjects.

• If your teen is at the most problematic end of the spectrum for any of the five dimensions, this book will guide you in making some changes to help your child, but it especially will tell you how urgently you need to act and how you can find the most appropriate health care resources for your teen. I firmly believe that solving eating- and weight-related problems is a matter of teamwork among health care providers, parents, and teens. An experienced and empathic health care provider can bring objectivity and calm to a turbulent situation and, through early involvement, can often keep problems from doing serious harm, but he or she cannot do it without you. Health care providers tell me time and time again that family support and healthy role modeling are essential for successful treatment.

Our Susceptible Teens

What We Know about Causes and Contributing Factors

"What causes weight-related problems?" This may be the most pressing question that parents ask me. And it is often followed by the questions, "How do I know if my child is at risk?" or "Why my child?" Because most of us suspect we're at fault when a child ends up overweight, develops an eating disorder, or shows signs of having a poor body image. After all, feeding our kids is one of our primary responsibilities as parents. One 16-year-old we interviewed related the painful memory of a woman who years earlier had brazenly asked her mother—right in front of her daughter—how she could have let her little girl get so fat. Parents who ask me what causes weight-related problems want to be assured that they're not to blame. I have no hesitation assuring them they're not. It's much more complicated than that.

Research has clearly shown that obesity and eating disorders are caused by many factors that interact with each other. One negative remark or television show, in and of itself, will not cause an eating disorder. A few too many stops at McDonald's in lieu of home-cooked dinners will not, by themselves, lead to a lifetime of overweight. Teens function within families and peer groups, which operate within institutions such as schools and work sites, which are located in communities. All of these systems are influenced by broader social norms and public policies. There are different levels of influence, and factors from within each of the levels play a role in the onset of weight-related problems, as shown in the following diagram, inspired by a model created by Dr. Urie Bronfenbrenner.

The factors affecting weight-related issues can be pictured as a series of concentric circles, each representing a sphere of influence:

- *Individual* characteristics such as eating behaviors, personality, and genetics.
- *Family* factors such as weight talk at home and family meal patterns.
- *Peer* influences such as peer dieting norms and peer participation in sports.
- *School* and other institutional factors such as weight-teasing policies within schools and school lunch food.
- *Community* factors such as opportunities for teens to get involved in different activities and community safety.
- *Societal* factors such as media influences and gender role expectations.

Not only do all these different factors play a role in causing an eating-related problem or affording your teenager protection from it, but each layer of influences affects the others as well, as shown by the arrows pointing in both directions. As a parent, you have an influence on your teens and their development, but surely your teens also influence how you respond to them. The kinds of foods you buy and serve at meals have an influence on what your children eat. But your children's food preferences also influence the food you serve. School policies regarding vending machines can influence soda pop intake among teens, but reactions by teens and their parents to the presence of vending machines can have an impact on what is sold.

The fact that things are so intertwined can make changes challenging. Parents may naturally be more concerned about the eating patterns of a child who clearly has a genetic disposition toward obesity and therefore increase their monitoring of what the child eats. All well and good, except that this vigilance can, although unintended, disrupt a child's food regulation skills and lead to increased overeating. If you've spent a good part of your life worrying about your own weight and trying different diets, this, no doubt, has had an influence on your teen's weight concerns and eating behaviors. In turn, her own concerns may have affected the types of conversations she's had with her peers about weight-related issues and even the types of magazines she reads. If family meals haven't been the norm for you, your teen may have gotten in the habit of going out with friends to grab a bite, which may discourage you further from bothering to cook. I hope that reading this book will urge you to consider making some positive changes in your own attitudes and behaviors, but as with any change, it won't happen overnight. Keep your expectations reasonable and hang in there.

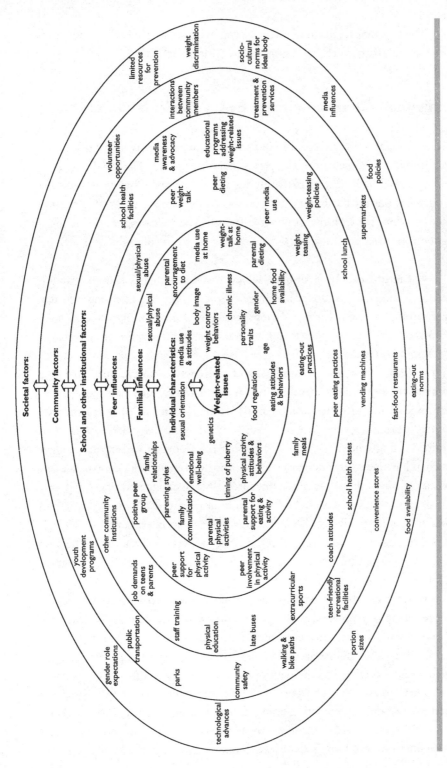

A holistic and integrated approach for understanding factors causing weight-related problems: Spheres of influence.

25

The best first step is to know what you're up against in each sphere of influence, and, fortunately, the research has a lot to tell us.

Individual Characteristics: Every Child Is Different

The individual characteristics of your teenager that can play a role in causing weight-related problems run the gamut from fixed traits like gender and genetics to modifiable factors like attitudes and behaviors. Obviously, you can't do much about the fixed traits, but you should be aware of their influence and how they interact with the modifiable factors. The following are a few highlights from the research:

- **Dieting can be a double whammy.** Research has shown that unhealthy dieting can go too far and increase a teen's risk for an eating disorder, or it can lead to binge eating, placing a teenager at risk for obesity. As I'll explain more fully in Chapter 6, it's a good idea to discourage your teenager from going on a diet.
- **"Eat when you're hungry and stop when you're full" may be some of the best advice around.** In a study on adults, the risk of obesity was six times greater in white women and 15 times greater in African American women who ate beyond satiation every day, as compared with women who stopped eating when they were full. Eating in response to emotional hunger (such as loneliness) and external stimuli (imagine seeing a big chocolate cake) instead of physical hunger can contribute to binge eating and obesity. It may also be followed by purging and lead to bulimia nervosa. Not paying attention to the internal signs of hunger is also a part of anorexia nervosa, although in this case teens avoid eating in response to hunger. Some ideas for helping teens to eat when hungry and stop when full, in a supersized food environment, are presented in Chapter 9.
- **Poor emotional well-being can contribute to different types of weight-related problems, while personality traits may be more selective.** Through fairly complicated and highly variable routes depending on other factors, both low self-esteem and depression can increase your teenager's risk for unhealthy dieting and the development of an eating disorder or for overeating and excessive weight gain. Body dissatisfaction is one of the strongest predictors of unhealthy dieting and eating disorders; it is also strongly correlated with obesity, although it is probably more an effect of obesity than a cause. Interestingly, having an obsessive–compulsive or perfectionist personal-

ity increases the risk for eating disorders, yet doesn't seem to be related at all to obesity. In a large study, those with anorexia scored nearly twice as high on a perfectionism scale as a comparison group. This may be due to a desire to perfect dieting or, more broadly, to a desire to perfect oneself. Likewise, sexual orientation seems to be related to eating disorders (with higher rates among homosexual boys than heterosexual boys) but not to obesity. While it is unclear why this is so, interactions between personality factors, identity formation, and social norms regarding attractiveness may be contributing elements. We need to maintain close contact with our teens so that we're tuned in to their emotions.

- **Where exercise is concerned, anything but moderation can cause a problem.** Regular and enjoyable physical activity can help protect your teen from developing any type of weight-related problem. But too little physical activity can contribute to the onset of obesity, and excessive exercise can contribute to the development of an eating disorder (see Chapter 5). Most of us send our kids off happily, even proudly, when they say they're going for a run or heading for the gym or meeting a friend to play tennis. But are they doing this three times a day? Are they spending more time at the gym than on homework and social life combined?

- **Puberty is hard enough—but it's even harder for teens going through it differently.** Girls who develop early and are larger than their peers may get attention they aren't ready for and may be at increased risk for body dissatisfaction and unhealthy weight control behaviors. Furthermore, hormonal differences in these girls can contribute to obesity. Boys have an advantage over girls in that what they get with maturation—height and increased muscle mass—is deemed desirable. But this leaves boys who develop later than their peers vulnerable to painful teasing and exclusion. There's not much you can do to modify your teen's rate of physical maturation, but you probably can pay extra attention to whether developing at a different pace than the other kids has made your teen feel uncomfortably self-conscious, acknowledge the difficulties your teen may be facing, and reassure your child that he or she is normal.

| **what you can do** | → Acknowledge how difficult it can be to be different from one's peers, but reassure your teens that they are normal and that things will even out. Although it seems some- |
| PROVIDE TEENS WHO DEVELOP AT A DIFFERENT PACE WITH ADDITIONAL SUPPORT | |

what obvious, they need to be reassured.

→ Make use of outside resources to reinforce this message. Your teen may need to hear from your pediatrician that the changes he is experiencing are normal.

➜ Buy a book for your child such as *Growing and Changing: A Handbook for Pre-Teens* or *The Teenage Body Book*, both by Kathy McCoy and Charles Wibblesman (see Resources for these and other titles).

➜ Show your teens pictures of extended family members and point out physical characteristics that carry over different generations. This can help in recognizing what is and is not under their control and in establishing a sense of pride in characteristics that may set them apart from their peers and link them to their extended family, whether these characteristics are related to developmental pace or permanent traits. Be sure to discuss positive traits related to the appearance, personality, and/or life achievement of extended family members with whom they have similarities.

➜ Even if your teens are developing more quickly (or more slowly) than their peers, do what you can to help them feel special about the changes in their bodies. See page 30 for ideas on welcoming changes, such as the onset of menstruation.

➜ Be there to listen. Remember, sometimes all you need to do is provide support without trying to fix the problem.

Of course, every situation is different, and you know your children better than I do. I have a friend who took the bold step of inviting some of the kids who were teasing her middle school son about his height over to her house for pizza, so that they could get to know him better. I never would have thought of that idea . . . but in this case it was appropriate.

• **We're not bound by our genes, but they certainly play a role.** In fact, genetic predispositions, currently being researched, appear to play a role in both eating disorders and obesity (see box on facing page). Individuals with a mother or sister who has suffered from an eating disorder are twelve times more likely than people without a family history to develop anorexia nervosa and four times more likely to develop bulimia nervosa. Forty percent of overweight toddlers with at least one overweight parent remain overweight as young adults, as compared with only 8% of overweight toddlers whose parents are not overweight. Studies have also shown that the identical twin of someone who has an eating disorder or is overweight is more likely to have the same problem than a nonidentical twin or other sibling.

• **Being a girl may expose a teen to greater risk for eating disorders,**

but when it comes to excess weight, boys and girls are equal. Girls are nine times more likely to have eating disorders than boys, but the risk for obesity does not differ by gender at all in teens. This is probably due to greater social pressures on girls to be thin and, as a result, the rates of body dissatisfaction and dieting that are twice as high in girls as in boys. It may also be due to a greater sensitivity of girls to interpersonal conflicts (for example, in the family) and a greater tendency to internalize rather than externalize distress. This means that there may be a dual pathway to the higher prevalence of eating disorders among girls than among boys.

- **Age counts: That's why this book is about teenagers.** Adolescence brings many physical, psychological, and social changes. Major challenges include dealing with a rapidly changing body, finding one's identity, separating from one's parents, becoming more autonomous, and developing different types of peer relationships.

During early adolescence (ages 11–14), the physical changes of puberty have an impact on how teens view themselves and how others react to them. It's normal for teens of this age to feel some stress. But being teased about physical changes or, certainly, being sexually violated can have devastating effects on their self-esteem, body image, and resulting eating patterns. Late adolescence (ages 18–21) is another important transitional period, in this case forcing teens to deal with problems, often without their family's support, take on additional responsibilities (such as feeding themselves), and make tough decisions about their future as adults. It's not surprising, therefore, that during early and late adolescence teens tend to be more aware of their bodies and more sensitive to comments by others and are at higher risk for eating- and weight-related problems. Add to this the fact that it's easy to keep eating at the same rate after the adolescent growth spurt has ended and thereby gain

GENETICS OR ENVIRONMENT?

Genes for traits such as perfectionism or anxiety may increase one's risk for anorexia nervosa and genes for traits such as low metabolism or appetite regulation may increase the risk for obesity, in the presence of social-environmental factors such as pressures to be thin or the availability of excessive food. Dr. Cindy Bulik, who conducts genetic research on eating disorders, says, "Genetics load the gun, but environmental factors pull the trigger." Family history can help determine whether your teen is genetically predisposed to a weight-related problem. Look at your teen's environment to determine the risk for gene expression.

weight. Or the fact that when teens start becoming more autonomous and eating more on their own, they often choose food that is cheap, filling, and high in calories.

what you can do
HELP YOUR MATURING TEEN TO WELCOME CHANGE

As much as possible, we want to help our teens rejoice in the changes that are occurring in their bodies. For example, when our daughters begin menstruating, it's important to help them see this as a positive sign. Different families deal with the onset of menstruation differently, but some type of celebration can be helpful, such as taking your daughter out for lunch, buying her a small present, or somehow welcoming her into the world of women in your family and/or community. Dr. Linda Smolak, a developmental psychologist who works in eating disorder prevention, talks about the importance of "normalizing" menstruation (for example, don't hide tampons in the bottom of the shopping cart when you buy them). When her daughter began menstruating, she told her daughter that she had now joined the larger sisterhood of women along with Queen Elizabeth and many other famous women.

Family Counts!

I don't know about you, but there are days when it seems to me as though I'm not a major player in my teens' lives anymore. Yet research clearly shows that family counts quite a bit, even though teens don't always show it and peer influence is increasing.

- **Communication between parents and teens is key.** Talking and listening allows us to learn more about what's going on in the different spheres of influence surrounding our teens. Studies have shown that teens who feel that their parents care about them and that they can talk to their parents about important issues are at much lower risk for an array of problems . . . including disordered eating behaviors.
- **The example you set matters tremendously.** In one research study, we found that the main family factors that distinguished teens who used unhealthy weight control behaviors from those who did not were family meal

patterns and negative weight-related comments by family members. When family meals occurred on a fairly regular basis and family members did not make negative weight-related comments, girls were far less likely to use unhealthy weight control behaviors. The same applies to obesity. Home environments that reinforce social pressures to overeat and underexercise will increase children's risk for obesity. In contrast, children are less likely to be overweight when raised in homes that aim to filter out these pressures, when parents model healthy eating and activity, make healthy food choices available, prepare regular family meals, and provide opportunities for physical activity. Believe me, I know it's difficult to do all this, and so do your kids. Those we interviewed said they knew a lot of parents are away from home during the day and really pressed for time and that kids eat fast food on their way home from school because it's the easiest way for them to fill the gap left by the stay-at-home moms of yore. The solutions I offer later take into account all the obstacles we're up against in today's rushed world—no false promises of quick fixes.

• **Adopting an authoritative, instead of an authoritarian, parenting style helps.** Research suggests that an *authoritative* parenting style, defined by lots of affection coupled with a reasonable amount of expectations and structure, is the most effective for adolescent development overall and for preventing weight-related problems specifically. An authoritative style, by the way, also avoids exerting psychological control over your kids, such as using guilt to get them to "eat right." Less effective parenting styles for teens are an *authoritarian* style (lots of expectations without lots of affection), a *permissive* style (lots of affection but not enough expectations or structure), and an *unengaged* style (neither affection nor expectations). Many of us don't fit exactly into one style, but may have elements of different styles. When it comes to being an authoritative parent, with regard to sensitive topics such as our teens' eating and weight, things are often easier said than done; thus, we'll be coming back to how to do this throughout this book.

• **Sexual or physical abuse exacts a toll in the arena of weight-related problems too.** Sexual or physical abuse from family, friends, or strangers can greatly increase the risk of an eating disorder. In a national survey of 6,500 teenagers in the United States, 18% of the girls and 12% of the boys reported that they had been either sexually or physically abused. Girls who had been sexually and physically abused were at four times the risk for binge–purge behaviors (eating a lot of food and then making oneself vomit or taking laxatives), and teenage boys were at eight times the risk, in comparison

IS YOUR PARENTING STYLE A POSITIVE FACTOR FOR PREVENTING WEIGHT-RELATED PROBLEMS?

Research suggests it's important to *be responsive* to your children's dietary needs and food preferences when purchasing and preparing foods (without going overboard), *have expectations* regarding family meal routines (such as telling your kids they need to show up), and *not try to control* what and how much your children eat through comments that are meant to be helpful but can often be interpreted differently by a sensitive teen ("You're not going to eat another chocolate, are you?").

If you want to find out more about your own parenting style, complete the brief survey at *www.shouldertoshoulderminnesota.org.*

with teens who had not experienced any abuse. Teens who had experienced abuse and had not talked about it with anyone were at greater risk for binge–purge behaviors. So, if you think your child may have been abused, it is extremely important that you talk with him or her and do all you can to get the teenager to meet with a psychologist or other health care provider. For some individuals who have been abused, obesity is a solution for avoiding future sexual encounters or food may be used to deal with hidden pain. Fortunately, for the vast majority of overweight individuals, however, abuse is not an issue.

Teens and Their Friends

Scientific research has confirmed what you've seen for yourself: Peer influences can either increase or decrease your teenager's risk for weight-related problems (See Chapter 4).

First, the negatives:

• **Where there's fat talk, there's dieting.** Fat talk ("I look so fat." "No you don't; I look even fatter") can seem like the proverbial broken record if you listen in on a group of teenage girls. It's not harmless. Kids who have made this subject a part of their everyday conversation often diet too.

• **When there's teasing, weight-related problems may follow.** Being teased or otherwise mistreated because of their weight doesn't just hurt kids' feelings. Teasing by peers tends to expose teenagers to a higher risk of disordered eating behaviors, which, in turn, may increase the risk of eating disorders and obesity.

- **Teens resemble their friends on weight-related issues.** Does your teen belong to a peer group in which body dissatisfaction and dieting are the norm? We don't really know whether teens change their attitudes to match those of their friends or if teens pick friends with similar attitudes, but research shows that you'd be wise to keep your eyes and ears open to see what your teens' friends are up to.

Now for the positives:

- **Positive behaviors are shared too.** The fact that teens resemble their friends can go both ways. For example, one teen we interviewed talked about how teens will often go along with the crowd; if her friends wanted to walk somewhere, she'd walk with them—otherwise she'd take the car.
- **And so are positive attitudes.** Research shows that girls with a high level of body satisfaction are more likely to have friends who don't diet but who do care about "being fit and exercising."
- **Teens provide support for each other.** Peers can help prevent their friends from engaging in unhealthy weight control behavior, can provide support during recovery from eating disorders, and can help their friends feel good about themselves even if overweight. One girl we interviewed who struggles with her weight said it's who she is as a person that her friends care about; they see her as "big," not "fat." Although we often get caught up in talking about negative peer influences, we need to remember the important positive role that peers play in our teens' lives.

School and Other Institutions Where Teenagers Spend a Lot of Time

Our kids spend a big chunk of their day at school, and some spend a significant amount of time at jobs, especially during the summer. Do you know whether these environments are having a positive or a negative effect on your teen's weight-related attitude and behavior?

- **Some schools promote healthy eating at lunch and even offer good breakfast and after-school options, but many also rely on vending** machines and "à la carte" foods for extra income. These offerings aren't regulated by national nutritional guidelines the way the school lunches are supposed to be, and we don't need a research study to know that making soda pop available at lunch can't be doing our kids any good.

• **Health classes always address nutrition, but most don't address the broad array of weight-related problems effectively or treat the delicacies of weight-related concerns in teens with the necessary sensitivity.** For example, assessments of body composition, including percent body fat, which are done with good intentions, can have detrimental consequences for an already sensitive teen.

• **Phys ed and after-school sports have upsides and downsides.** Most schools don't require physical education classes every year in high school, and some schools are even talking about eliminating phys ed requirements altogether because of budget constraints. Questions are also being raised about whether students are active enough during gym classes, whether enough time is devoted to activities that can be done for life, and whether the classes meet the needs of kids who don't feel comfortable with their bodies. As to after-school sports, fewer and fewer kids participate as time goes on and interscholastic sports get more competitive. Facilities like basketball courts, fields, and pools usually end up being for the exclusive use of teams. And even if your child joins a team, can your family get him or her to and from practices and games if the school doesn't offer transportation?

what you can do
PARENT ACTIVISM CAN MAKE A DIFFERENCE

Parent advocacy work has led some school districts to refuse to make contracts with soft drink companies. As a busy parent, you may feel that you don't have the time, energy, or know-how to bring about changes in your children's school environment. But small actions, such as calling or sending a note to the school principal or a school board member about vending machine food choices or after-school transportation problems can make a difference, particularly if taken by more than one parent. At the very least, if you know what you're up against, you can take countermeasures at home, such as making sure your kids eat a good breakfast before they leave the house in the morning, buying some healthy snack foods for them to put in their lockers, providing transportation to team practices, showing up at games, and looking for other outlets for physical activity if the school offerings just don't work for your teen.

Community Factors: Where You Live Makes a Difference

Think about your own community. What features make it easy for your teens to be physically active, make healthy food choices, or, more generally, make some smart behavioral choices? What about your community hinders any interest your teen may have in engaging in these behaviors?

- Is it safe for your teen to go out biking or for a walk?
- Are there recreation centers or other facilities that are teen-friendly?
- Are high-quality fruits and vegetables available at your local grocery store?
- What types of restaurants are there in your neighborhood?
- Is there a fast-food restaurant or a convenience store in close proximity to your home or your child's school?
- Do your children have relationships with people in your community? Are there other adults to whom your children can turn if they need to speak with someone other than a parent? (Research has shown that caring adults, other than parents, can make a difference in a child's life with weight-related and any other problems.)
- Are there youth groups that foster positive youth development?

Research is beginning to explore the role of the community in encouraging obesity, so data should be available in the future. In the meantime, I'm not suggesting you relocate if your community doesn't offer a lot of positive preventive resources, just that you know what you're up against so you can take countermeasures as necessary at home.

Societal Factors: Pushing Fat but Rewarding Thin

Our teens are surrounded by mixed messages and negative societal influences. Teens whom I've interviewed admit that if they didn't have the Internet or a TV, they might be out there getting exercise. One said that his monthly computer use added up to several 24-hour days. As Chapter 4 explains, media influences are enormous . . . and so are portion sizes. For now, suffice it to say that I see our social environment as one that "pushes fat but rewards thin," encouraging us to overeat and be sedentary, yet stay unrealistically thin and muscular.

A TOXIC ENVIRONMENT

Dr. Kelly Brownell, a leading figure in eating disorder and obesity prevention, describes our environment as one that is "toxic" in terms of its impact on weight-related disorders: "It is difficult to imagine an environment more effective than ours for producing nearly universal body dissatisfaction, preoccupation with eating and weight, clinical cases of eating disorders, and obesity."

Is Your Teen at Risk?

Now that you've got the big picture on the numerous factors that can contribute to weight-related problems, it's time to put it to work in determining the status of your own teenager. On the following pages you'll find worksheets to help you identify the factors within the different spheres of influence that are at work in your child's life and what you can do to offset any negative factors. I'm not asking you to do this alone. I've done the exercise with one of my children. You may find it helpful to take a peek at what I've done.

Maya, my 15-year-old daughter, agreed to serve as an example on condition that I didn't make up anything. As you read the following evaluation of Maya, refer to the filled-in worksheets that I did (on pp. 40–42). Maya appears to be at low risk for developing a severe weight-related problem. But, like most teenage girls, she is at moderate risk for the less problematic eating-, activity-, and weight-related issues that were also shown on the spectrum in Chapter 1. At the individual level, Maya is involved in some sports that could increase her sensitivity to weight and overall appearance. In gymnastics, she needs to wear a leotard, and, clearly, attention is given to overall appearance during competitions. Furthermore, appearance in general is pretty important to her, and she spends a fair amount of time deciding what to wear to school, how to do her hair, and so forth. She also spends a good amount of time watching those teen "reality" shows on TV that seem populated with photogenic people with nothing but appearance- and sex-related concerns. Maya is also involved in a number of activities that don't emphasize appearance; she volunteers, goes to youth activities at our local community center, and attends a summer camp that works on enhancing ideals related to social justice. Furthermore, she belongs to a teen dance group that includes kids of all shapes and sizes.

Family and peer factors also serve as risk and protective factors. Within our family there is a fair amount of sensitivity to weight-related issues, and my kids know that certain comments are just not acceptable. I've always worried

IS YOUR TEEN AT RISK FOR A WEIGHT-RELATED PROBLEM? WHAT ARE THE RISK AND PROTECTIVE FACTORS?

Individual characteristics
What are some individual characteristics that might increase your child's risk?

What are some individual protective factors that might decrease your child's risk?

Familial factors
What are some family factors that might increase your child's risk?

What are some family factors that might decrease your child's risk?

Peer influences
What are some peer influences that might increase your child's risk?

What are some peer protective factors that might decrease your child's risk?

School and institutional factors
What are some institutional factors that increase your child's risk?

What are some institutional protective factors that decrease your child's risk?

Community factors
What are some community factors that increase your child's risk?

What are some community protective factors that decrease your child's risk?

Societal factors
What are some societal factors that increase your child's risk?

What are some societal protective factors that decrease your child's risk?

TAKING FIRST STEPS TOWARD CHANGE: WHAT ARE YOUR THOUGHTS?

Based on the information in the preceding worksheet, would you rate your teen's risk for a weight-related problem as none, low, moderate, high, very high, currently present? Which weight-related problems seem to be of most concern?

What is one risk factor that you would like to change or work toward minimizing its impact on your teen? How might you go about doing this?

What is one protective factor that you would like to reinforce? How might you go about doing this?

that since I work in eating disorders prevention, my teens might choose to act out by engaging in disordered eating behaviors. Maya's friends engage in some fat talk, but overall they seem to have positive body attitudes and healthy eating and physical activity patterns.

It was great to think about Maya's school. My sense is that there really is acceptance of diversity among students—regarding appearance, dress, race, and so forth (and Maya confirmed that when we discussed the worksheet). This was not the case in a previous school district where we lived, and it was something we looked for when we moved. But, at the broader societal level, I found that most factors have the potential to increase her risk for an array of weight-related problems.

Through this process of examining specific risk and protective factors, I was able to begin thinking about areas for change: Check out the atmosphere of the gymnastics team and the coach's attitude, keep lines of communication open so that Maya will discuss arising concerns with me, eat meals together more often, talk with Maya and her friends about dealing with fat talk, discuss healthy food options at school and provide her with healthy snacks to keep in her locker, and actually watch some of those awful television shows to get a better idea of what she is watching and add my two cents' worth.

This process helped me think about my daughter's risk for developing a weight-related problem, identify factors that seem to be helpful and harmful, and think about actions I can take to decrease her risk.

After doing this worksheet, I showed it to Maya to make sure it accurately reflected the situation. This also provided us with an opportunity to talk about some of these issues and for her to provide me with more information. I encourage you to do the same. The more we talk, the more we learn, and the more we know what to say and do.

YOUR TURN . . .

Now, to fill in the blanks for your own teen, take a look at each of the spheres of influence and ask yourself about specific protective and risk factors. Does your teen seem to be at low, moderate, or high risk for a weight-related problem? What type of weight-related problem? What are some of the influencing factors that you want to reinforce? What are some of the risk factors that you identified? What are your initial thoughts on working to modify these risk factors or decrease their influence on your teen? Write down some of your ideas on the first worksheet provided here.

If you feel comfortable doing so, consider showing this worksheet to your teen to get a discussion going about some of the issues in his or her life. Or just ask your teens about specific influencing factors that you may not know about and that are relatively easy to bring up for discussion. For example, ask your teens if they talk with their friends about dieting and whether any of their friends have eating disorders.

A first step toward change is recognizing what the issues are. Some say that once you've recognized the issues, you're more than halfway there. Start thinking about how you can work toward modifying some of the risk factors you've identified. Pick one for starters. Give yourself credit for the protective factors you've identified, and think about ways to further enhance them even further.

ASSESSING RISK AND PROTECTIVE FACTORS FOR A WEIGHT-RELATED PROBLEM IN MY DAUGHTER

Individual characteristics

What are some individual characteristics that might increase your child's risk?

Female. Watches a fair amount of television with thin actors. Likes to read magazines for teen girls. Concerned about appearance. Short height bothers her. Involved in gymnastics and dance. Doesn't do a lot of unstructured activities such as walking.

What are some individual protective factors that might decrease your child's risk?

Low genetic disposition for obesity and eating disorders. Does some sports that don't emphasize weight—such as lacrosse and soccer. Although she dances and does gymnastics, it's not at an elite level. Has pretty regular meal habits. Doesn't diet.

Family factors

What are some family influences that might increase your child's risk?

Chaotic family schedules can interfere with family meals. Computer in bedroom can decrease family interactions and decrease physical activity. Eat out a fair amount. Father loves to watch sports events on television. Mother works in eating disorder prevention—therefore always has fear that she will "rebel" in this area.

What are some family protective factors that might decrease your child's risk?

Role modeling of healthy and "normal" eating and physical activity by parents (mother is a nutritionist and father is a physical education teacher). No encouragement to diet or making negative weight comments. Overall good family relations. Parenting practices that encourage autonomy but provide structure. Home availability of a variety of foods.

Peer influences

What are some peer influences that might increase your child's risk?

Some fat talk among peers.

What are some peer protective factors that might decrease your child's risk?

Supportive friends who generally have healthy behaviors.   (cont.)

School and institutional factors

What are some institutional factors that increase your child's risk?

Parents' jobs can interfere with family time and food preparation time. At school there are unhealthy choices in vending machines and fast food options for lunch. Limited late buses after sports means she needs to get rides home from family or friends.

What are some institutional protective factors that decrease your child's risk?

Enjoyable physical education program at school. Opportunities for participation in school sports even if not star. Health classes address nutrition and eating disorders. School norms are supportive of diversity in appearance.

Community factors

What are some community factors that increase your child's risk?

Very limited public transportation (need parents for rides). No lights in neighborhood. McDonald's across from school.

What are some community protective factors that decrease your child's risk?

Youth program with teen volunteer opportunities at local community center. Local supermarkets with good produce. Community safety is high. Nearby walking paths. Nice relations with neighbors.

Societal factors

What are some societal factors that increase your child's risk?

Constant exposure to media images that promote thin body as ideal. Gender expectations to be attractive and conform to certain look. Sociocultural norm emphasizing importance of thinness. Technological changes that make it easy to be inactive. Excessive food availability and large portion sizes.

What are some societal protective factors that decrease your child's risk?

Food policies such as national guidelines for the type of food that can be served as regular school lunch. Some restrictions on movies that teens her age can see. Availability of fruits and vegetables and other healthy food options. But it seems as if most societal factors work to increase risk for obesity, unhealthy dieting, and eating disorders!

TAKING FIRST STEPS TOWARD CHANGE: WHAT I LEARNED ABOUT MY DAUGHTER

Based on the information, would you rate your teen's risk for a weight-related problem as none, low, moderate, high, very high, currently present? Which weight-related problems seem to be of most concern?

Low for weight-related concerns at most problematic end of spectrum such as obesity, clinical eating disorders, anorexia athletica, binge eating disorder, and severe body dissatisfaction. Moderate risk for less severe weight-related problems such as dieting, moderate body dissatisfaction, and erratic eating behaviors.

What is one risk factor that you would like to change or work toward minimizing its impact on your teen? How might you go about doing this?

I am concerned about media influences on her body image. In the past I have involved her in some of the media training activities that I have done for younger children, and I am going to look for other opportunities to do that again, since I think it is empowering for her. I am also going to watch, with her, a few of the television shows that she tends to watch, to get a better idea of what's going on in them so that we can talk about some of the underlying messages.

What is one protective factor that you would like to reinforce? How might you go about doing this?

Involvement in non-appearance-related activities. She has just gotten involved in a youth group that plans social justice activities, such as an upcoming summit on volunteer activities for teens within our community. I am going to do my best to support my daughter's involvement in activities of this type through positive reinforcement and providing transportation as much as possible.

"How can we protect our teens when society pushes fat but promotes thin?"

If your children were completing a survey, would they say that you "diet"? If you're not sure, ask. Then think about what you can do to get to view you as a "healthy eater" rather than a "dieter." A lot of their ressions come from the way you talk about things. Watching your ght? Have a juicy slice of watermelon instead of a piece of pecan pie dessert; just don't say something like "I'd love the pie, but I'd better , because I'm dieting."

KE-HOME MESSAGE

void unhealthy, noticeable behaviors altogether, such as fasting, skipping heals, or drastic food restrictions. I'd be very careful with the low-carb diets hat were all the rage as this book went to press (just one example of the extreme regimens that foster unhealthy attitudes by labeling whole categories of food as "bad"), since it would be pretty hard for your teen not to notice that you're eating your burger with a slice of bacon instead of a bun. If you're watching your weight, adopt eating and activity behaviors that you would like your children to emulate, and pay attention to the way you talk about them. If you say anything at all, put the focus on health—not on weight.

Even if you stop at the gym on your way home from work every day, this good example may be lost on your teen if he or she isn't there. Consider going to the gym together and look for ways to get physically active at home,

As to food choices, the conclusions are obvious: If you want your teens to drink milk at dinner, give up your diet cola or coffee and pour a glass of milk for yourself too.

What You Say Also Matters

As suggested earlier, it's not just what you do but also what you say that matters. In fact, when it comes to promoting good eating and activity behaviors, *this may be one of those rare instances when what you say counts even more than what you do*. Parents often encourage their children to diet because of genuine concern for their children. They want their kids to avoid all the physical and psychosocial complications of being obese in our society. The problem is it just doesn't work. Encouraging your children to diet is likely to lead to the use of unhealthy weight control behaviors. Ironically, these behaviors can lead to

3

Parents Matter (a Lot)

I said it in Chapter 2, and I meant it: If your teenager has a weight-related problem, it's not your fault. But as the news makes you increasingly aware of the rise in obesity and eating disorders in American teens, you can't help becoming more conscious of your own weight-related issues. You've probably already asked yourself whether your daughter has taken your offhanded comments about needing to go on a diet much more seriously than you ever intended. Maybe you've wondered whether your son's fascination with bodybuilding magazines is healthy and whether it's a result of watching his father and older brother compete over muscle mass at the gym.

Of course, it's never that simple. But the research described in Chapter 2 has important lessons for us: Our kids do watch and listen to us. They also watch and listen to their friends, as well as videos, movies, the Internet, and all the purveyors of giant sandwiches, mega-fries, and mac-and-cheese. And it all has an effect on what and how much they eat, their physical activity habits, and how good they feel about themselves. Since your influence is more powerful than you may have realized, why not use it to offset the negative messages your teenagers are getting everywhere else?

Step 1 is always self-awareness. To exercise your power, you need to be fully cognizant of your own weight-related issues and the subtle as well as direct messages you might be sending to your kids.

What Your Kids See You Doing Makes a Difference

Research studies have shown a strong association between more extreme weight control behaviors in parents and similar behaviors in their teens. The research shows that if your children see you skipping meals, going on a crash diet, or fasting, they're more likely to do the same. We see this in practice as well as in research studies. Many of the eating disorder professionals I've interviewed have told me that if there's one piece of advice for parents they'd like to see in this book, it's "Don't diet. Model behaviors you want your children to adopt."

Whether the same association exists between more moderate weight control measures in parents and unhealthy weight control behaviors in teens is harder to say. "Dieting" means different things to different people. Depending on how questions on dieting behaviors are asked, the answers can vary considerably and may not accurately represent any one type of practice. In Project EAT, 25% of boys who perceived that their mothers "don't diet at all" engaged in unhealthy weight control behaviors, as compared with 49% of boys whose mothers "diet a lot." And 50% of girls who perceived that their mothers "don't diet at all" engaged in unhealthy weight control behaviors as compared with 72% of girls whose mothers "diet a lot." Interestingly, nearly identical associations were found with fathers' dieting behaviors: 25% of boys who perceived that their fathers "don't diet at all" engaged in unhealthy weight control behaviors, as compared with 52% of boys whose fathers "diet a lot." And 54% of girls who perceived that their fathers "don't diet at all" engaged in unhealthy weight control behaviors, as compared with 70% of girls whose fathers "diet a lot."

The factor that makes the difference may be whether your teens really notice your behavior. Teenagers may adopt their parents' behavior in cases of crash dieting and fasting because they can hardly avoid noticing when a parent doesn't show up at the dinner table, or shows up but either eats nothing or eats something different from everyone else. A review of the scientific literature shows that studies using parental reports of their own dieting behaviors show weaker associations with their teens' dieting behaviors than studies in which teens give their perceptions about their parents' behaviors. Although parental reports of their own behaviors may be more accurate, teen reports of their parents' behaviors necessitate that the teens have actually noticed the behaviors.

Girls who are going through puberty and experiencing changes in their bodies are more likely than others to diet in the same way as their mothers. This is not surprising, since during these transitional periods teens are more physically self-

conscious and may be more attuned to what thei[...] trol their own body weights. Interestingly, one [...] mother–daughter pairs who were at greatest risk[...] tudes and practices were those who were simultane[...] ductive transitions likely to lead to weight gain. A [...] weight because of puberty while a mother may be ga[...] pregnancies, menopause, or the side effects of hormo[...] This process may make mother and daughter more likel[...] curring in each other and to be more sensitive to each[...]

As with dieting, whether teens exercise more when their [...] on whether they see their parents in action. Much of the ph[...] assessed in research studies is activity that we do without o[...] witness it. Again, studies that ask teens to report their perce[...] ents' physical activity and sedentary behaviors tend to show[...] tions with the teens' behaviors than studies using parental rep[...] activity levels.

What about food choices? Do teens eat like their parents?[...] we found that *teenagers whose parents report eating more fruits, [...] dairy foods were also more likely to eat more of these foods.* For examp[...] parents who ate four or more dairy servings a day ate two-thirds [...] more than teens whose parents didn't eat any dairy foods. (Th[...] sound like a lot to you, but that's because we're talking about popu[...] ages.) One of the reasons for the stronger parent–teen association [...] than for exercise is that teens probably have more opportunities to [...] parents are eating than what kind of exercise they are doing.

what you can do	When both you and your teen ar[...]
TAKE ADVANTAGE OF YOUR TEEN'S INTEREST	ing through physical changes (for [...] ample, during puberty, pregnancy, [...] menopause), your teen may be part[...]

ularly tuned in to how you are handling the changes. Try to demonstra[...] acceptance of these changes and talk about them in a positive way. I'v[...] found it helpful to talk about how neat it is that our bodies change in ac[...] cordance with our needs at different stages of life. I also talk about how [...] natural it is for body shapes to change over time. I try not to make nega[...] tive comments about getting wrinkles or gaining a few pounds. Model [...] healthy behaviors, such as eating breakfast and staying active, and avoid un[...] healthy weight control behaviors, especially at this time.

binge eating, which can actually cause weight gain (see Chapter 6). A second group of research studies showed that teenagers are disturbingly compliant when parents encourage them to diet. Even worse, *a simple comment by a parent about weight or dieting meant to be helpful can often be misconstrued by a vulnerable teenager*, and kids often report being hurt when a parent tells them they need to lose weight.

In a well-designed Australian study of 369 10th-grade girls and their parents, parents were asked how often they encouraged their daughter to lose weight and whether they would like their daughter to be thinner. The girls were asked about their dieting behaviors, whether their parents encouraged them to diet, and if they felt that their parents criticized their weight. Parental encouragement to diet and teens' perceptions of parental criticism of their weight were associated with teens restricting their diets, unhealthy measures like skipping meals, fasting, and crash diets, and symptoms of bulimia nervosa. The associations were stronger with *daughters' perceptions* of parental encouragement than with *parental reports* of encouragement, just as they were for parents' dieting behavior.

Interestingly, in this study many of the parents were not even aware that their daughters were using unhealthy weight control behaviors. The vast majority of parents of girls who were fasting, crash dieting, vomiting, or using laxatives or diuretics did not know their teens were dieting or thought they were dieting about the right amount. These findings demonstrate how important it is for us to check with our teens and avoid making assumptions about what they may or may not be doing.

what you can do
THINK ABOUT THOSE INNOCUOUS STATEMENTS WE ALL MAKE AND HOW THEY COULD BE TAKEN

You may think you're offering helpful advice. But, because teens are so sensitive to their bodies, they may be hearing something different. Comments like these can easily be taken out of context: "Are you sure you want a second helping?" "Have you put on a bit of weight?" "The soccer coach might consider you more seriously for varsity next year if you lost a little weight to give your speed and agility a boost." "I just read about a new diet that looks great; it might interest you." Try to avoid talking about dieting or making comments about weight at home. If you're concerned about a weight gain in your teen, wait for him or her to bring up the topic . . . and then ask what you can do to help. (More on what to do when they bring up the topic in Chapter 14.)

Parents Matter

49

WHO MATTERS MOST—MOTHERS OR FATHERS?

Drs. Susan Paxton and Eleanor Wertheim of Australia have extensive research and clinical experience with teens. In an interview in Melbourne in 2003, they said both parents matter. Mothers probably have a larger impact on their children than fathers, since mothers tend to diet more, have a greater role in food preparation, and may talk to their teens more about food and weight. But comments made somewhat innocently by fathers (and older brothers) can be very disturbing to teenage girls. Girls with eating disorders often recall a hurtful weight-related comment serving as a dieting trigger.

Boys may take encouragement to diet even more to heart than girls. In Project EAT, 51% of boys who were encouraged by their mothers to diet for weight control reported unhealthy weight control behaviors, as compared with 22% who were not encouraged. Even more frightening, 10% of boys who were encouraged by their mothers to diet used extreme weight control behaviors such as vomiting, laxatives, diuretics, and diet pills, as compared with only 1% of other boys. Finally, and somewhat ironically, 15% of boys whose mothers encouraged them to diet reported binge eating, as compared with only 2% of other boys.

TAKE-HOME MESSAGE

Don't encourage your daughter or son to diet, and certainly don't suggest a mother–daughter diet the way many mothers used to do. Instead, encourage your child to try some alternative lifestyle behaviors that can be implemented on a long-term basis—see Chapters 5 (physical activity) and 8 (healthy eating). If you want your kids to be more physically active, you may have to make it easier for them to do so, not only by verbally encouraging them but also by driving them to the game or going for a run with them.

what you can do
PAY ATTENTION TO THE MESSAGES YOUR TEEN GETS FROM FRIENDS

In Project EAT, teens who reported that their parents and friends were dieting *and* that their parents encouraged them to diet were very likely to be dissatisfied with their bodies and using unhealthy weight control behaviors. If you know your teenager's friends are dieting and using fat talk, make a special effort to avoid negative weight-related comments. Remember the spheres of influence in

Chapter 2; often our role as parents is to counteract (and certainly not reinforce) negative pressures coming from other spheres of influence, such as peers.

Is There Room for Change?

I would love you to come away from this book with a positive body image, a total lack of any prejudice against fat people, and a decision to stop dieting and instead employ healthy eating and physical activity behaviors on a regular basis. But I also recognize how hard this can be to achieve. As a first step, modify the behaviors most likely to impact your teens: those that are (1) are noticed by your teens and (2) are directed toward them (for good or bad).

Do any of these behaviors sound familiar?

Samia flops onto her mother's bed as Mom gets dressed for a formal dinner out. She watches as her mother frowns at her reflection in the mirror and says, "I feel so bloated today." She asks Samia how she looks in her outfit, "What do you think? Does it make me look thinner?"

Nick often goes to the gym with his father. One evening, after showering, his dad looks in the mirror and mutters, "All this working out and I just can't get rid of this stomach. I wonder if it's worth the time!"

Ruth is constantly trying to get her children to watch less television, but her husband loves to flop down in front of the TV after a long day at his construction job. During his favorite sports seasons, he can get stuck there for hours. Ruth isn't happy about the mixed messages her children are getting.

By now I'm sure you can see that the kids in these families are watching their parents model less than optimal behaviors and attitudes toward weight-related issues. If you're starting to realize that you may be doing the same kind of thing, the good news is that the behaviors most likely to impact your teens may be the easiest ones to change. Some examples:

- It may be easier to stop making negative comments about your body or others' in front of your teen than to actually improve your body image or drastically change your ingrained weight-related attitudes.
- You may not totally be able and willing to give up drinking diet soda,

but you don't need to drink it every night for dinner when eating with your children.

- You may not be willing to give up all dieting, but you should stop any diet plan that interferes with normal family meals.
- You may not be willing to totally stop weighing yourself, but you could get rid of your scale and weigh yourself only at the gym.

MAKING A COMMITMENT TO TAKE SMALL STEPS TOWARD CHANGE

For each of the four questions that follow, pick at least one behavior that you're willing to adopt to be a positive role model. Short of ideas? Check out the list at the end of this chapter.

- What *positive self-care behaviors* do you already use? Choose at least one that you're going to make sure you do this week (for example, keep on eating salad at dinner; say nice things to myself when I look in the mirror; continue to walk three times a week).

  _____

  _____

  _____

- What can you do to *make sure that your teen notices* your positive behaviors? Choose at least one thing you can do that you'll make sure your teen notices this week (for example, drink milk when my kids are looking; when my daughter is in the room, look in the mirror and something nice about myself; announce, "I'm going for a walk").

  _____

  _____

  _____

- What are some behaviors of yours related to weight control, physical activity, or eating that you do *not* want your teen to adopt? Choose one that you're going to stop this week (for example, stop skipping breakfast; stop buying diet books; stop talking about weight).

  _____

  _____

  _____

- What are some things that you can say to *enhance your teen's body image?* Choose at least one to say this week (for example, compliment your teen on something she is wearing, avoid saying anything aimed at changing her weight or appearance).

_____

_____

_____

Ideas for Changing Your Own Eating-, Activity-, and Weight-Related Behaviors: Be a Positive Role Model for Your Children

- Eat breakfast with your kids in the morning.
- Eat a piece of fruit after dinner.
- Tell your family that you've given up dieting and instead are focusing on lifestyle changes.
- Give up dieting and begin to focus on lifestyle changes.
- Eat salad at dinner.
- Offer other family members salad at dinner.
- Go for a walk in the evening and invite your teen to go with you. Go again the next evening.
- Take a look in the mirror and identify five things you like about yourself.
- Give yourself compliments, in front of your children, on your appearance. Practice saying, "I think I look pretty good in this new outfit."
- Give yourself compliments, in front of your children, not related to your appearance. Tell your children about a major accomplishment at work today.
- Talk about the new bike path you've discovered or how much fun your jazz class is.
- Ask your teens how you can help them be more physically active. Then follow through.
- Prepare a shopping list before going grocery shopping. Ask your kids about healthy foods they'd like for the week.
- When you look in the mirror, make sure to take note of at least one positive.
- Don't make negative comments about your weight and appearance in front of your children. Resist the urge—it may be hard at first, but it is so important!

- Don't make negative comments about your weight and appearance in front of anyone.
- When you see family members and friends you haven't seen for a while, avoid making comments on their weight such as "You've lost (or gained) weight."
- If you're concerned about your teen's weight, don't encourage him to diet. Instead start making some changes in the home food environment and be there when he's ready to talk.
- Compliment your teens on their appearance. Then say it again.
- Praise your teens for their accomplishments. Then say it again. And again.
- Plan family outings that involve physical activity.
- Don't say anything negative about your body or appearance for a whole day. Then do it for another day.
- If you have an urge to binge, wait 10 minutes and either go for a walk, take a shower, or call a friend.
- Buy bottled water instead of soda pop.
- Buy an outfit that fits you now and praise yourself in it.
- Read magazines that make you feel good about yourself. Avoid the others.
- Get physical for fun. Go for a walk in nature or sign up for a dance class.
- Reassure others who are concerned about their weight without putting yourself down.

By the Way, We're in This Together . . .

I wish I could say that as a result of so many years of working in the areas of eating disorder and obesity prevention I'm a perfect role model for my four kids and never get down on myself after getting on the scale, say anything I later regret, or deliver mixed messages. I can't. I'd be lying if I told you that I never wished that my legs were a few inches longer and my butt a few inches narrower. And there have been times when I've commented on someone's appearance and my kids have laid into me: "I can't believe *you* said that! Isn't that a bit hypocritical?!" What I *can* say is that through my work in this area I've made some enormous changes. I can honestly say that most of the time when I look in the mirror I make a point of noticing the positives and that in general I tend to make healthy food choices, engage in "normal" eating patterns, and do some physical activity each week. I never "diet"; instead I make gradual modifications in my eating and physical activity patterns at times. I can honestly say that I've learned to appreciate the beauty in different people's body shapes and sizes, regardless of whether they fit the typical societal ideals. Only on a rare occasion do I make a comment about someone's weight, whether positive or negative. And it's even rarer that I make negative weight-related comments about myself or about others around my children. This is why I think taking a few steps toward changing any negative behavior that is likely to influence our teens is worth the trouble. But it's an ongoing journey, and one that we'll continue to take together throughout this book.

4

Friends, Fashions, and Fads

*I*t comes at them from every direction: the pressure to be thin, to look fit, to be "healthy." Their friends are on diets or working out every day after school. Photos of pop idols depict a lean, hard-body ideal. Jokes and scorn are heaped on anyone who doesn't measure up (or down). Gyms are everywhere, diet books abound, and there's simply no excuse for being overweight.

Except, of course, for the fast-food joints on every corner, the allure of ever more graphically sophisticated video games, and enticements to go with the larger burgers, fries, pizza, and soda since you get more for your money.

The competing pressures to stay thin, but to sit still and eat more, are undeniable. The question is how strong the influences of peers, media, and other social factors really are on our teens and what we can do to tip the balance from negative to positive.

The answer begins with knowing exactly what pressures are coming to bear on your teenager when you're not there to witness them.

Jenny sits at the end of a long cafeteria table eating the school lunch. Her considerably shorter and skinnier friends are picking at their food; they avoid the pizza, which they say is way too greasy to eat, and eat only the salad and bread stick. One of them is talking about how fat she's been feeling and how she's skipped breakfast, will eat a small lunch and dinner, and won't eat anything between meals. Jenny's famished, but as her friend goes on, she puts down the pizza and covers it with her napkin.

After lunch Jenny has phys ed, where they're beginning a two-week swimming unit. Jenny gets into her swimsuit, which she hasn't worn since last summer, and finds it a bit tight. Glancing in the mirror, she thinks her stomach looks incredibly bloated after the pizza at lunch, and she sees that her suit is creeping up her "enormous" thighs. Reluctantly, she heads for the pool, where her teacher makes some comments about how teenagers have been getting fatter over the past two decades because of their low levels of physical activity. Jenny feels as though he's looking directly at her.

After school, she takes a TV break before getting to her homework; while watching television, she can't stop comparing her own body shape and size to those of the actors. By the time her mom gets home from work, she's feeling pretty lousy; she keeps thinking about how she looks as compared with the thinner girls at school and those on that TV show. What her mother sees when she walks in the door is a girl with a sullen look on her face, sprawled out on the family room floor, looking like she's never planning to move from that spot. Tentatively, she asks Jenny how her day has been, and when she gets nothing but a grunt in reply, she says, "Well, you might feel better if you got out and got some fresh air." Her daughter responds by jumping up and stomping toward the front door. As the sound of the slammed door reverberates through the house, Jenny's mother wonders what she's done wrong now.

Sound familiar? I can't count the number of times I've been an unwilling actor in a scene like this. Like Jenny's mother, I've made what I thought was a sensible suggestion without having any idea of what my son or daughter had been through that day and how my well-intentioned advice would be received. Jenny's mother saw that her daughter looked down and thought that getting outside might help, as it often does when *she* feels stressed or has the blues. Because of all the input Jenny has gotten during the day, she heard her mother's advice like this: "Well, you wouldn't feel so bad if you weren't fat from sitting around in front of the TV all the time."

Many parents of teens, whether they're trying to help an overweight teenager make changes or prevent unhealthy habits in the first place, feel that their role is to give advice—about the nutritional content of food, the benefits of dieting, why not to take another helping of potatoes, the difficulty of taking the weight off later, the importance of exercise, and so on. This may be appropriate in certain situations. But if your teen is surrounded by thinner peers at school who are constantly talking about how fat they feel and discussing their diets over lunch, she's probably aware of all this and already feeling the pressure. And you may never hear about all the small occurrences during the day that have hurt her feelings and her self-image.

The moral of this story is that the more you know about the pressures your teenager is under all day, the less you'll have to rely on assumptions that may just earn you the disdain of your teen and close off those all-important lines of communication. In Chapter 13 I'll give you lots of ideas for talking—and, most especially, listening—about these sensitive topics with your teens in a way that will encourage them to open up, and maybe even listen to whatever advice you do want to impart. In the meantime, though, knowing what the research has shown us about all these outside forces can arm you with a better understanding of what your kids may be going through—and what you might be able to do to help.

Friends and Other Peers: The Good and the Not So Good

Sure, the term *bad influence* fits some of your teenager's peers. And, yes, expecting nothing but wisdom to be passed from one adolescent to another is a little like hoping your cat will house-train your dog. But the influences of your child's friends aren't all negative. Teens are more likely to go out for a high school sport when their friends do too. And as any high school girl will tell you, all the parental pep talk in the world can't hold a candle to the positive reinforcement of a group of supportive friends. A girl in one of our studies remembered with crystal clarity how her friends jumped in with fierce loyalty when she felt so bad about her looks that she didn't want to go to school. Proclaiming her a beautiful person and lifting her mood and self-image, these girls had a positive impact that lasted for several days and was never forgotten. Likewise, the understanding that comes from confiding in those who share your experience offers valuable stress relief, which all teens need. If it doesn't always come with great advice . . . well, that's where we adults come in. I hope some of the information that follows will help you filter out the undesirable messages without demonizing your kids' friends, which rarely accomplishes anything other than driving your teenagers away from you and toward the friends with a vengeance.

CLIQUES: SHARING CLOTHES, DIETS, AND BODY ATTITUDES

The research confirms our suspicions that friends can have a strong influence on teens' weight-related attitudes and behaviors. Dr. Susan Paxton and her colleagues came up with a terrific way to identify cliques and then explore the weight-related attitudes and behaviors the members shared. They asked each girl in their study to identify up to five of her best friends from a list of all the girls in the school; they then designated girls as belonging to a friendship group when each of them named the others. That is, if Dana wrote down Marla and Laura, and Marla wrote down Dana and Laura, and Laura wrote down Dana and Marla, they were viewed as a clique. Not only did the study find strong similarities in body image attitudes, dieting, and extreme weight control practices within each clique, but girls with higher levels of body image concerns and weight loss behaviors reported (1) talking more about weight loss and dieting with their friends, (2) comparing their bodies more often with others, and (3) being teased more often by their friends about weight and shape. These findings suggest that observing your daughter's friends may tell you a lot about your own teenager's attitudes toward weight-related issues, even if she is not very outspoken about them with you.

FAT TALK: A CODE YOU CAN BREAK

Typical conversation overheard by a fly on the wall in any high school girls' restroom:

ROLLIE: I feel so fat.

KATHY: You feel fat? I feel really fat. These pants make my butt look huge.

ROLLIE: Don't you love what Alison is wearing today? She's gorgeous. She's so thin—she's really lucky. No wonder she's so popular.

KATHY: I should have bought the black pants instead of these khaki ones; they would have made me look thinner.

What exactly is going on in this conversation? What is Rollie looking for when she says she feels fat? What do the girls really mean when they say that they "feel" fat? Why does Rollie choose to compare herself to Alison, a "popular" thin girl?

When teenagers, particularly teenage girls, engage in fat talk, they're often looking for reassurance. Rollie may say she feels fat because she'd like her friend to let her know she looks okay. Her friend does try to reassure her, but because she does so by saying she also feels fat, they end up sharing the misery more than any positive support.

What does it mean to "feel" fat? Author Sandra Friedman (*When Girls*

Feel Fat and other titles; see Resources) correctly states that fat is not a feeling. If we don't challenge the statement, though, we can hardly argue with the logic of the teenager's response, which might be to go on a diet. Unfortunately, dieting won't erase the feeling, because *being* fat is not the issue. Solutions that *will* resolve the uncomfortable feeling will depend on what the feeling is: insecurity, depression, loneliness, or the like. Therefore, if your teenage daughter says, "I feel fat," the answer may not be to suggest a new diet for becoming thin (or to support a diet she is already on), but rather to explore why she feels the way she does.

Rollie and Kathy's fat talk moved seamlessly from their own bodies to another, more admirable one. This phenomenon has been called the "body comparison trap." It's not hard to understand how comparing themselves with the thinner Alison and attributing her popularity to her thinness could only exacerbate the girls' dissatisfaction with themselves. Yet we all seem to fall into the comparison trap, if not about weight and shape, then about some other characteristic, such as wealth or fame or family stability. Teens are more susceptible because of their limited life experiences, their developing sense of identity, and their greater tendency to compare themselves with others and be influenced by their peers. Research shows that teens who tend to compare their bodies with others often make comparisons with those who have "better" bodies than they do and end up with greater body dissatisfaction.

HELP YOUR TEEN DEAL WITH FAT TALK AND AVOID GETTING CAUGHT IN THE BODY COMPARISON TRAP

So, how do we help our teenagers deal constructively with fat talk and avoid getting caught in the body comparison trap? First, we teach them how to respond when they hear fat talk. Let's assume Daniella walks into the restroom and overhears Rollie and Kathy immersed in fat talk. If Daniella is like most girls, she'll probably join in: "If you guys think you look fat, take a look at me. You're both thinner than me." This type of remark probably would succeed in bonding the girls together, but it wouldn't do anything to reassure Rollie and Kathy about their appearance. Daniella might even come away with some new self-doubts that she wasn't feeling earlier. But that's not how it has to go. She could say something like this: "We're always comparing ourselves to those few girls that are all skinny and stuff, and that makes us feel bad about how we look. It's dumb and we should stop doing it. You guys look really pretty just the way you are . . . plus you're a lot of fun to hang out with, and that's what really counts." In this scenario, Daniella reassures her friends that they look great, talks about the importance of not making only "upward" comparisons with others, and brings up nonappearance strengths of the girls. With just a few sentences, Daniella bonds with the other girls and provides the needed reassurance for her friends and herself. You can model this kind of response for your teens.

Here are a few other ideas for countering fat talk and avoiding the trap:

- Rent the movie *Real Women Have Curves* (or a similar one) for your teenage daughter and her friends, order in pizza, and get the girls to talk about their reactions to the movie and to begin to think about alternative ways of viewing their bodies. This movie depicts a girl dealing with body image issues and a mother who is putting pressure on her to lose weight. It's a fun movie that deals with important topics for adolescent girls.

- Ask your teenage daughter (or son) if her friends ever talk about "feeling" fat and what that means. Ask your daughter what might be some ways of responding when other kids say they feel fat, other than saying that she also feels fat. Tell her about the body comparison trap and share your own experiences—how you also tend to make comparisons with those who are "better" than you in one way or another and how you're trying to stop doing this since it makes you feel worse about yourself instead of better.

- Keep in mind that your teen is likely to be comparing herself to the "cream of the crop," whether it be her body shape, style of dress, or intelligence. Remind her of her strengths and provide positive reassurance. Teens need to hear this from you again and again.

- Take a look at the kinds of behaviors you might inadvertently be modeling for your teens. When friends tell you they feel fat, instead of saying you also feel fat or have gained weight, comment on how great you think your friends look, without getting down on yourself.

what you can do
LOOK FOR OPPORTUNITIES TO TALK ABOUT THIS STUFF

Think about one topic you could bring up this evening at dinner, or while driving around in the car, to encourage your teen to feel proud of her body and question social norms that aren't working in her best interest. Talking about this kind of stuff isn't always easy, so I try to look for opportunities to have these discussions. On a recent trip to New York, my daughter and I were lucky enough to see the Broadway play *Hairspray*, which addresses both weightism and racism in a teen-friendly and very entertaining manner. One evening at home, I watched the movie *Mona Lisa Smile* with my daughter, which allowed for a brief conversation about how things have changed for women over time in regard to expectations and roles. . . . I got in a few sentences before my daughter let me know that I shouldn't get too carried away.

Teasing: It's Not Okay to Make Fun of Someone's Weight

Anyone who has ever been overweight and was called "fat" knows that this kind of insult hurts. The current research reveals how deeply ugly weightism can be. I fervently hope that being aware of the full impact of this form of discrimination will move all of us to establish zero tolerance for weightism.

WEIGHTISM: THE LAST OF THE SOCIALLY ACCEPTABLE "ISMS"

Weightism may be the last form of socially acceptable stigmatization tolerated in our society. Why is it tolerated? My experience is that many people don't really take weight teasing seriously. People may not even realize that they've made weight-related comments that have hurt others or that they've been the victim of weightism. They may not realize how common weight stigmatization is and how detrimental it can be for a teenager. This is compounded by the fact that many people see weightism as different from race or sex discrimination, since they view weight as controllable. They view individuals as being responsible for their body shapes and sizes and thus feel that weightism is more tolerable than other *isms*.

My research team conducted in-depth individual interviews with 50 overweight adolescents to learn about their experiences with weight stigmatization. In the interviews with African American teens, one-third said they had been treated unfairly because of their weight, one-third because of their race, and one-third because of both their race and their weight. It was very painful to hear the last group describe this double prejudice: distrusted because of a prejudice that linked skin color with criminal predilections and disdained because of a prejudice that linked obesity with poor hygiene and lack of character. These kids knew that racism was wrong, but it wasn't always clear to them that the same was true of weightism. Some of their comments suggested that size discrimination is more socially acceptable and less socially suppressed in our society than racial discrimination. They sometimes gave the impression that they thought they should find it more acceptable too. We also sensed that these teens may have had more opportunities for bonding and for developing a sense of pride in being African American than in being overweight. Although there are fat acceptance groups that aim to empower individuals of all shapes and sizes, these groups and their messages do not seem to be reaching teens.

In fact, the sense that mistreatment of overweight individuals is somehow acceptable emerged among the entire group of teens who were interviewed. When asked to generalize about their experience, some of the teens initially said they hadn't been mistreated because of their weight. Yet they then began to talk about being treated differently by the boys at school or to remember hurtful comments from parents or being singled out for being "fat" in elementary school. Even more disturbing, these teens frequently made excuses for those who had treated them badly, referring to the abuse as "just normal" playground behavior or justifying it by saying "they were just joking around," "they didn't mean it," or "they were just trying to be helpful." In some cases the teens may not have wanted to admit that they are mistreated because of their weight; in others it seemed as if the teens began to recognize that the way they had been treated was not okay only as we continued to talk.

WEIGHT TEASING: HOW COMMON IS IT?

Ignoring weight stigmatization keeps the world at large from realizing how widespread it is. Yet throughout the course of the interviews, experiences of mistreatment because of their weight were described by virtually all of the teens. Of the 50 teens we interviewed, 48 described hurtful comments that were made to them or about them and/or differential treatment or rejection because of their weight. The discrimination ranged from being called "fatso" or "pig" directly, to receiving comments couched as helpful, such as "How come you're eating that?" or "Don't be so lazy," to social exclusion or outright rejection. (See more on what these teens shared with us in Chapter 14.)

As a result of the earlier study, we decided to explore this phenomenon in a larger, more representative sample of teens and included questions on weight teasing in the Project EAT survey. As you can see in the following table, it wasn't just overweight teens who were teased but underweight teens too—anyone who deviated from the average.

Friends, Fashions, and Fads

	Percentages of teens who report being teased about their weight by their peers	
	Girls	Boys
Underweight teens	48%	41%
Average-weight teens	21%	14%
Moderately overweight teens	31%	26%
Overweight teens	63%	58%

These data are drawn from Neumark-Sztainer D, Falkner N, Story M, Perry C, Hannan PJ, Mulert S. Weight-teasing among adolescents: Correlations with weight status and disordered eating behaviors. *International Journal of Obesity.* 2002; **26**: 123–131.

WEIGHT TEASING: DOES IT REALLY MATTER?

Yes. It matters a lot. Teens who are teased about their weight may feel bad about it and react either by taking extreme measures to lose weight or by overeating to make themselves feel better. Project EAT found that teenage girls and boys who are teased frequently about their weight are twice as likely to use unhealthy weight control behaviors and two to three times as likely to binge eat as teens who are not teased about their weight. Weight teasing may, therefore, have implications for both eating disorders and obesity. Indeed, teens in treatment for eating disorders often recall experiences in which they were teased about their weight, which may have triggered their initial dieting behaviors. And some overweight individuals binge eat as a way of coping with difficult emotional and social situations such as being teased or treated badly.

Even more alarming, we found that teens who were teased about their weight were at risk for a broad array of concerns including low body satisfaction, low self-esteem, depressive symptoms, and suicidal thoughts and attempts. Teens who were teased by both peers and family members were at greatest risk. Let me share some numbers with you to demonstrate how strong these findings were and to impress upon you how serious weight teasing can be for teens:

- In girls, low self-esteem was found among 16% of the girls who were not teased about their weight, 25% of girls who were teased by either peers or family members, and 37% of girls who were teased by both peers and family members.
- Thoughts about suicide were reported by 25% of the girls who were

not teased about their weight, 36% of girls who were teased by peers, 43% of girls who were teased by family members, and 51% of girls who were teased by both peers and family members. Half of the girls who were teased by both peers and family members about their weight have had suicidal thoughts!

- Similar patterns, although not quite as strong, were found among teenage boys who were teased about their weight.

Do these figures leave any doubt about the impact of weight teasing on emotional well-being? Sometimes the comments of one individual can mean more than statistics on thousands. One girl described it as trying to put her self-esteem back together bit by bit but constantly being "cut down" until eventually she had no self-esteem and sometimes just broke down. As a result, she said, "Sometimes you close yourself out of the world." In Chapter 14, you'll read more about the experience of weight stigmatization in the overweight teen's world and will be left with no doubt that weight stigmatization exists—and matters.

SPEAKING OUT AGAINST WEIGHT STIGMATIZATION

It seems pretty obvious that we need to act now to eliminate weight teasing from our homes, schools, and communities. Easier said than done, I know. Many of us don't like to make a scene when we encounter weightism personally. Recently, on a flight to Los Angeles, I heard a man behind me say loudly about the empty middle seat in his row, "I sure hope some fat chick doesn't come and sit here. Then she's going to want to take up the armrest." I spent the rest of the flight fuming and building myself up to say something by thinking of all the instances throughout history when speaking out might have made a difference. So, at the end of the trip, I finally said I thought his earlier comment had been inappropriate and that although he might be disturbed if a large person sat next to him, he should think how uncomfortable a large person would feel having to squeeze into a tiny middle seat on a plane. I was flabbergasted when he flew into a blaming rage about how he too would like to stay up until two in the morning eating chocolate cake and ice cream!

Maybe what I said couldn't possibly have gotten through to him. On the other hand, he just might think twice before saying like that similar again. Furthermore, all of the people around us heard the conversation, and perhaps they too will avoid making such comments and even feel empowered to speak out if they hear something similar. I *can* say that speaking out made me realize that weightism truly does exist and that we can speak out against it. We *have* to speak out against it.

This does not mean that I am promoting obesity. It means that I think people of all shapes and sizes need to be treated with respect and that we all need to avoid making assumptions about and judging overweight individuals' behaviors. For health reasons, I strongly believe we should do everything we can to encourage our kids to maintain a healthy weight. But we need to recognize that there are many obstacles to doing so, including a genetic predisposition toward a higher body weight, impediments to going out for a walk or bike ride, and living in a household in which it is hard for a parent to be at home to prepare healthy meals.

We can work to promote a healthy body weight in ourselves and in our children while respecting those whose weight deviates from the norm. We need to speak out against weightism, for the sake of overweight individuals and for the sake of all individuals who, regardless of their size, obsess about their weight for fear that they, too, will be the target of weight-related mistreatment. Teens who hear others being teased about their weight are bound to fear that they might be teased as well, regardless of their current weight.

So, what can you do?

1. Pay attention to what you say. You may not realize you're saying anything hurtful . . . but your teen may be taking your comments quite differently. Many of the teens we interviewed talked about how painful they found "helpful" remarks from their parents or "jokes" from others. I myself am guilty. I remember the shock I felt when one of my sons told me I had teased him about being too thin, and he remembered my comment years later. Ask your teens if you've said anything that has bothered them about their weight. Then make every effort to change.

2. Make negative weight-related comments unacceptable at home. Despite my earlier slipup, my family now knows that weight-related comments won't be tolerated. Your teens should feel that home is a safe zone, no matter how rough it is for them outside.

3. Don't laugh at weight-related jokes. You don't have to laugh. Let the person doing the joking feel uncomfortable when no one laughs.

4. Role model antiweightist attitudes and behaviors. Avoid making any comments about other people's weight, particularly comments that tie weight to personal character (for example, fat and lazy). Stick up for others who are victims of weightism.

5. Support your kids in the face of weight mistreatment. You may be tempted to suggest ways for your child to lose weight as a strategy to avoid being the victim of weight teasing. This is very natural, as you want to help your child to be happier. Please resist doing this, since it feeds into the premise that somehow your child is responsible for the weight teasing. Provide support if your child reveals he's been teased about his weight or excluded from a friendship or a school team because of his weight. Save the advice on weight control for a different conversation.

6. Talk with your teens about how they can react if they hear others being teased about their weight. Brainstorm ideas with your teens on how they can refuse to participate in a conversation about weight or how to speak up against weightism. Ask them questions to give them an opportunity to think about possible responses: "What would you do if kids were planning to ask a fat classmate for her phone number as a joke? Would you join in the fun? Or would you tell them it was a stupid idea? Would you warn the girl or her friends?" Ask them how they would feel in such a situation. Acknowledge how difficult it can be not to buy in to such talk and to take a stand against it. Most teens won't find it easy to take such a stand. But if you appeal to their sense of fairness and justice, they might surprise you. Many teens are more receptive to addressing the problem of weight teasing if it is framed as weightism, a form of discrimination comparable to sexism or racism.

7. Let your teens know they don't have to put up with any form of weight teasing. Ideas for dealing with weight stigmatization, through the four R's (Recognition, Readiness, Reaction, and Repair), are discussed in Chapter 14.

8. Reach out beyond your family. Find out what weight-teasing policies your teen's school has established. If you don't find them satisfactory, get involved in working toward the implementation of clear guidelines as to what is and is not acceptable. Suggest that similar guidelines for the consequences of teasing about racial issues or bullying be applied to weight teasing. We're currently working on the issue of teasing with staff and students at a local elementary school. Teasing emerged as an issue in a needs assessment done with children and parents, and we brought this information to the attention of the school staff. Now we're working to make changes through in-school programs, after-school activities, and policy decisions. The program is called "Very Important Kids," (VIK) and the idea is that since kids are special they should be respected and shouldn't be teased. Some of the activities include choosing library books that address teasing, having the children make antiteasing posters, getting the kids involved in developing consequences for kids who tease others, and having the students develop a school play that addresses issues such as body appreciation, respect, and teasing. For additional ideas on becoming an advocate for fighting weightism, see Margo Maine's book *Body Wars*. Another book, *Body Aloud!*, provides guidelines for setting up youth-led programs in schools or youth organizations to help teenage girls accept a wide diversity of body shapes and sizes. A wonderful website worth checking out for ideas on "boosting body image at any weight" is *www.bodypositive.com*. Additional ideas for reaching out beyond your family to fight weightism can be found on the Dads and Daughters website (*www.dadsanddaughters.org*). A teen-friendly site for promoting size acceptance is *www.size-acceptance.org/bbteens*. (See the Resources section at the end of the book for information on these resources and others.)

The Long Arm of the Media

Think about it:

- The U.S. federal government's largest nutrition education program for the general public (the 5 A Day program to promote fruits and vegetables) has an annual communications budget of about $3.6 million. In contrast, about $68 million is used just to promote M&Ms candies, and McDonald's spends about $1 billion annually on advertising and promotions. The total annual amount spent by the food industry on advertising and promotions: *$25 billion a year*. No wonder we're not eating enough fruits and veggies. For these and other shocking figures, check out the Center for Science in the Public Interest's website (*www.cspinet.org*).

- A study of the content of *Seventeen* magazine, perhaps the most widely distributed magazine for adolescent girls, found that consistently, over many years, the largest percentage of pages was devoted to articles about appearance.

- TV commercials almost exclusively show slim, healthy-looking people using whatever product is being advertised, including foods such as Big Macs, fries, soda pop, milkshakes, and huge restaurant portions of steak and potatoes or pasta.

At the same time, media advertisements promote foods that tend to be low in nutrients and high in calories. One teen said, "We're just bombarded

THE MEDIA AND MEN

In a study of the 10 most popular magazines commonly read by men and women, women's magazines had 10 times more articles related to dieting and weight loss than did the men's magazines. Men are targeted less often than women with messages about weight and appearance, and there is more diversity in what is acceptable for men in terms of age, size, skin, and appearance. However, the image of the lean and very muscular male is becoming more prominent in magazines.

An interesting study by Dr. Harrison Pope and his colleagues that examined 30 years of male action toys, including G.I. Joe figures and Star Wars characters, found that these toys have grown increasingly muscular over time. The earliest G.I. Joe (1964) has no visible abdominal muscles; his 1975 counterpart shows some abdominal definition; and the 1994 figures display the sharply rippled abdominals of an advanced bodybuilder. The authors concluded that "many modern figures display the physiques of advanced bodybuilders and some display levels of muscularity far exceeding the outer limits of actual human attainment." Thus, teenage boys who do not fit the lean and muscular ideal, or see themselves as fitting this ideal, are not immune to the media's impact on the way they perceive their own bodies. Boys may be dissatisfied with their bodies because they want to be thinner and/or because they want to be more muscular. In extreme cases, males who want to be bigger may develop "reverse anorexia" or extreme muscle dysmorphia, in which a desire to be larger can lead males to take their workouts to an unhealthy extreme.

One study found a significant increase in referrals of males to an eating disorder unit between 1984 and 1997, but it is not clear whether this reflected a greater prevalence of eating disorders among males or a greater willingness to seek treatment. Whether the media played a role in this increase is not known, but it is noteworthy that among those in treatment a higher percentage of males (37%) than females (13%) were "involved in an occupation or athletic team in which control of weight is important for good performance."

To date, less research has focused on males than on females, but watch for more research on media influences on teenage boys … and, in general, on trends in boys for body dissatisfaction, unhealthy weight control behaviors, muscle-enhancing supplements, anabolic steroids, and eating disorders.

on TV and stuff. We see all the celebrities eating things from McDonald's and Burger King. If they actually showed us that there were 51 grams of fat in a Big Mac, that would motivate me to eat healthy. I don't want to put that junk in my body." Just think about how many advertisements you see for fast-food restaurants and beer as compared with advertisements for fresh produce! Furthermore, media use such as television watching tends to be a sedentary activity. Through the promotion of foods high in calories and replacing physical activity with sedentary activity, media exposure and use may also be putting people at increased risk for binge eating, decreased physical activity, and obesity.

Can there be any doubt that media exposure and use (TV watching as an alternative to physical activity) may have implications for the broad spectrum of eating-, activity-, and weight-related concerns? Sometimes the impact is a simple and direct one. We see a TV ad for potato chips and French onion dip, and get up to grab something similar from the kitchen. Other times it's more complicated. Is your daughter destined to want to be as thin as the models portrayed in teen magazines or on television just because she's been exposed to these images? Will your son be doomed to steroid use if he watches movies starring actors sporting extreme muscle mass (which may not even be real)? Fortunately, some revealing research is helping us sort it all out:

FIJI GETS TV—AND WEIGHT ISSUES

Dr. Anne Becker and her colleagues happened to be in the right place at the right time to conduct a naturalistic experiment examining the impact of media messages. In 1995 she was in Fiji when television was introduced. She assessed the impact of television on the weight-related attitudes and behaviors of high school girls right then, as well as three years later:

- Vomiting for weight control purposes went from 0% to 11% among the girls over the three-year period following the introduction of television.
- High scores on an assessment of eating pathology (for example, unhealthy weight control behaviors) more than doubled during this period, increasing from 13% to 29%.
- Girls living in households with a television set were more than three times as likely to have high scores on this assessment of eating pathology.

In interviews that were carried out at the second assessment, the girls talked about how television had influenced them or their friends to feel differently about their body shape. The girls expressed admiration for television characters and a desire to emulate them by changing their hairstyles, clothes, or body shapes. They also talked about increased intergenerational tensions regarding the adoption of Western customs and expectations regarding an appropriate amount to eat.

This unusual study showed that not only did viewing thin characters on TV change girls' attitudes about how they should look, but so did their friends' responses to what they saw on TV. Girls were more likely to try to emulate television characters that their peers favored. Remember the concentric spheres of influence in Chapter 2? Here we see them at work in life, as the media and peers interact to influence teens' weight-related attitudes and behaviors.

NEWS FROM DOWN UNDER:
THE MEDIA ARE POWERFUL BUT NOT OMNIPOTENT

In an interview study with adolescent girls in Australia done by Dr. Eleanor Wertheim and her colleagues, girls revealed the many different ways the media influenced their body image:

- Seeing thin models in ads, on TV, and in magazines made them feel they weren't good enough, pretty enough, or thin enough.
- They got lots of dieting information from magazines.
- They were acutely aware that the fashions portrayed in the media were often unsuitable for bigger or even average-sized girls.
- The number of girls who said they felt a great deal of pressure to be thin from magazines and TV was higher than the number of girls reporting pressures to be thin from peers and family members.

The scientists' conclusions? First, that the girls perceived the media portrayal of the thin ideal as a major pressure to be thin. However, from the girls' remarks during the interviews, the authors also concluded that these media influences had been reinforced by a more immediate subculture that included peers and family. If friends and family can reinforce the messages the media deliver, the converse also ought to be true: They can weaken the impact by filtering out these messages and deemphasizing weight at home.

Project EAT compared teenage boys and girls who reported often reading magazine articles in which dieting or weight loss are discussed, with those who hardly ever read these articles, and found that:

- Girls who read articles on dieting or weight loss were six times more likely to engage in extremely unhealthy weight control behaviors, such as self-induced vomiting and use of laxatives, diet pills, and diuretics, than those who didn't.
- These girls were more likely to have lower self-esteem and lower body dissatisfaction and to be more depressed than girls who didn't read such articles.
- Boys who read the articles were at four times greater risk for extremely unhealthy weight control behaviors than boys who didn't.
- Boys who read the articles had lower self-esteem and were more depressed than boys who didn't. Associations with body dissatisfaction were apparent but not straightforward, suggesting a need for further exploration.

* * *

Strong associations between media use and unhealthy weight-related attitudes and behaviors were found in all three of these studies, even though they all used completely different research designs and were done in three different places in the world.

STRATEGIES FOR COUNTERACTING THE MEDIA'S NEGATIVE MESSAGES

Not everyone exposed to the media develops weight-related problems. What tips the balance? As you might guess, a lot depends on the prevalence of other negatives among the spheres of influence discussed in Chapter 2. If your daughter is already full of self-doubts about her appearance and tends to compare her body with others, for example, TV and magazines' portrayal of unrealistic body shapes is more likely to increase her body dissatisfaction and lead her to diet or overexercise. Look back at the worksheet you filled out in Chapter 2 to see how many negative factors exist in your daughter's life. The more you see, the more effort you'll want to put into the following strategies.

Strategy 1: Reduce Media Exposure

Let's start with television. In Project EAT we found that teenage girls watch an average of 18 hours of television or videos in a week and teenage boys watch an average of 20 hours. Teenagers reported spending more time watching television than reading and doing their homework (16 hours per week for girls and 13 hours per week for boys).

It may not be possible for you to get rid of your television. It sure wouldn't work in my house. But I challenge you to think about ways to decrease its use. You know your family better than I do; would any of the following ideas work in your home?

• Keep the TV out of your kids' rooms. Having a television in a bedroom increases its use and isolates your teenagers from the rest of the family. In interviews on family meals, some teens told us they take their food to their bedrooms and eat alone in front of the television. A research study on preschool children found that children with television sets in their rooms watched more television and were more than 30% more likely to be overweight than those without TVs in their rooms, even after taking into account other factors such as age, race, and mother's weight status. A study on middle school teens found that having a TV in one's bedroom was strongly correlated with increased TV viewing (and with decreased reading time). I realize that it might be difficult to yank a TV out of your kid's room if it is already there . . . but if you haven't allowed it yet, try not to give in on this one.

• Banish the TV from meals. Not only does watching TV during dinner increase everyone's exposure to negative messages, but it robs you of the chance to find out what's going on in your kids' lives. If what's going on in your teenager's life is a budding eating disorder, you'd want to know it, wouldn't you? You may not notice if all eyes are glued to the screen. Finally, watching TV means you pay less attention to what you're eating, which may mean you eat more than you really want or you simply fail to relish your meal, which is the way we're meant to experience our food.

• Turn the TV off the minute it's not getting the viewers' full attention. Some families leave the TV on as background noise. Even if no one is sitting in front of it constantly, TV's messages may continue to infiltrate our minds as we pass in and out of hearing range.

• Try listening to music instead of making TV the major source of evening relaxation. Or consider silence, conversation, or reading.

I urge you to take on the assignment of thinking of one way to decrease TV use in your own home. When we moved to our new house a few years ago, we purposely didn't put a television in our bedroom; this made a huge difference in the amount of late-night television that my husband and I watch. It also made it easier to stick by our principle of no televisions in children's bedrooms. This may not work for you, but something will.

What about other forms of media? TV is a big source of media in our society, but it sure isn't the only one. In fact, time spent on the computer and using the Internet surpasses television time for many teens. What can you do to decrease exposure that may have a detrimental impact on your teen?

- What magazines do you subscribe to? If your teen wants to subscribe to a teen magazine, check it out first to see if the positive messages outweigh the negatives.

- The computer can be an excellent resource, but in addition to keeping them immobile, it can expose teens to undesirable messages such as those at pro-anorexia sites, set up by individuals who have eating disorders. (For a further explanation of these sites, see *www.something-fishy.org*). Computer programs that allow you to restrict or monitor the sites your kids visit are available, or you can place computers in a room used by the family to allow for informal monitoring. Some parents figure their best bet is to talk with their kids about the dangers of these sites and tell their kids how to avoid unintentionally going to them. What works for you will depend on your own philosophy and your children's ages, among other factors. I use informal monitoring with my younger son and the "talk and hope" strategy with my older teens.

- What about movies? videos? music? Give some thought to what usually works in your family, based on your values, your kids' maturity, and practical matters.

Strategy 2: Teach Your Children to be a Critical Audience

Your teenagers are smart, and they don't like to be fooled. Show them that the media can't be counted on to convey the whole truth and nothing but the truth, and they'll become champion critics. Not only will this help them filter out the falsehoods and negatives on their own, but they're likely to spread their wiser viewpoint by sharing it with their friends.

There are many ways to get them started. Most of the following ideas were used in some form in the Free to Be Me program we ran for Girl Scouts ages 10–11. Our goal was to increase the girls' media literacy skills by increasing their awareness of media distortions and how media messages should be analyzed critically. I've adapted the ideas for home use here.

- Teenagers need to know that the beautiful models featured in magazines are not as they seem. Most images are modified by computer technologies to give the models smoother skin, leaner bodies, or more defined muscles. To help your teens avoid falling into the body comparison trap, let them know they're comparing themselves with a computer image, not a real person. Better yet, if someone in your house has some computer skills, you can play around with images on the computer. Using a program like Photoshop, you can manipulate pictures of family members to make them thinner, fatter, taller, and with smoother skin and different hair color. My son did this for us—very effective in getting the message across.

- Help your teenagers see how "ideal" body shapes have changed over time, particularly for women. Take a look at the beautiful, full-figured young women in Renoir's paintings. Remind your daughter that Marilyn Monroe, who was considered one of the great beauties of all time, was a size 12. Look at pictures of women from the "flapper" period, when it was considered stylish to be very flat and almost boyish. Ask her what she thinks about how Twiggy looks (first let her know who Twiggy is and the large impact she seems to have had on the current sizes of models). Today a more muscular, but very lean, body is viewed as attractive. Ask your teens, "Is it realistic for women to change their body shapes in line with the current fashion?"

- You can take the discussion a step further by looking at practices aimed at "improving" women's bodies over time in different cultures. Corsets were used to decrease the size of women's waists—to the point of breaking ribs. In fact, some young women had their lower ribs removed to allow for tighter corsets. Foot binding was used in China to prevent young girls' feet from growing too much; large feet could interfere with marriage prospects, so it was acceptable for a girl to have impaired mobility. What might future generations have to say about the types of weight-loss practices promoted in our time? What might they say about media messages that simultaneously discuss the dangers of obesity and eating disorders, yet promote overeating and a range of weight control strategies?

- For class projects in which they have a choice of topic, especially when they're supposed to choose a current controversy or issue, encourage your children to pick the media and its influence. Ideas include "The Media's Portrayal of Women over Time," "Media Messages to Children: Should There Be

Restrictions?" "Hidden Media Messages: What Are They Really Selling?" "Images of Men in the Media: How Are Things Changing?" "The Role of Media on Body Image: Does It Make a Difference?" and "Teens as Targets of the Media." My daughter is taking a speech class at high school, and just yesterday she asked me for ideas for a persuasive speech topic; I suggested some of these.

• Watch TV with your teens sometimes and talk about the kinds of messages that are being given directly and indirectly in the commercials and in the programs themselves. Use questions to see what your teens think: "Do you think the examples in those ads showing before-and-after weights are real?" "How do you think the girls who were excluded on *America's Top Ten Models* felt?" Avoid going overboard or they'll never want to watch a show with you again. It's another balancing act—you don't want to come off as being critical of your teen's choice of shows. A good guideline is to make one comment per show. You can also bring things up for discussion at a later point when you are in the car together or when your kids and their friends are sitting around the kitchen table having a snack.

• Talk back to the TV when you don't agree with the types of messages being given. "Yeah, right, my hair will look like that if I use your shampoo!" "What are you selling—the car or the woman?" "I'm sure you lost 25 pounds in 2 weeks without breaking a sweat." "Strange how they only show thin people eating burgers and drinking shakes; doesn't look like the crowd I see when I visit McDonald's." Be direct, make your viewpoint clear, use a bit of humor if you wish . . . but, again, don't go overboard so that your kids turn you off.

Strategy 3: Offset the Negative with the Positive

Use your teens' interest in media and their skills (which are often more advanced than ours) to your advantage. There are a lot of positives out there.

• If your teens are Internet-savvy, provide them with some of the teen-friendly Internet resources (see the Resources section at the end of the book). I just love the Girl Power site for younger girls (ages 9–13), which contains a lot of information on nutrition, body image, self-esteem, and growing up as a girl (*www.girlpower.gov*). Another great site for young girls is *www.forgirlsandtheirdreams.org*. The Body Positive site is great for older teens and provides a lot of information on improving body image and being an activist, taking steps toward changing media messages that lead to body dissatisfaction (*www.bodypositive.com*). Another site for older teens, aimed at inspiring critical analysis of media messages, is Mind on the Media (*www.motm.org*). Additional resources are listed at the end of this book, and the good thing is that many of these sites tend to be linked so that if your teen gets to one site, she will easily be able to get to others.

- Most of us are interested in getting our kids to read more. Magazines can provide good reading material, so find out what interests your teens and look for magazines that offer some decent messages. *New Moon* is an excellent choice for younger teenage girls who have pretty good reading skills. It is actually edited by a group of girls ages 8–14. I just checked out its website (*www.newmoon.org*), which describes some of the articles in the most recent edition; there's a quiz to find out "which musical instrument fits your personality," a story about a girl who visits the Auschwitz concentration camp, and an interview with Kathy Brier, who starred in *Hairspray* as a chubby girl who wants to act. This may give you a sense of how it differs from typical teenage girl magazines. *Teen Voices*, for older teenage girls, has a magazine and a website, and its motto is "Because you're more than just a pretty face." *Teen Voices Online* includes a regular feature in which teens speak out against ads (*www.teenvoices.com*). Don't forget about other magazines that might meet your teen's particular interests, such as *Sports Illustrated, Popular Science, National Geographic,* or *InTune.* What about magazines on dance, vegetarian cooking, or decorating? There is also an array of e-zines (electronic magazines) on topics such as photography, computers, and poetry.

- Look for television shows and movies with positive messages, and watch them together with your teens. This will provide your teens with positive messages and provide you with an opportunity to discuss them with your children. Some TV shows and movies that are of questionable educational value can become very educational when you view and discuss them together. This can also provide a venue for discussing topics that you might otherwise find difficult to bring up.

Strategy 4: Advocate for Change in Media Messages

Young children are being targeted with messages for candy, sugared cereal, and fast food during their television shows. Teen magazines contain articles about the dangers of eating disorders within the same issue that depicts extremely thin models and articles about weight loss. In advertisements directed at children and adults, females are portrayed as sexual objects. Even within schools, teens are being targeted with messages about soft drinks and foods high in fats and sugars. The list goes on and on. We can fight this by advocating for change in the types of messages that are given in the media and by restricting the entry of advertising into settings such as schools.

As parents, we have an important role to play in media advocacy work. It is absurd that our educational systems are dependent on soft drink companies and their advertisements within schools for needed revenue. As parents, we need to speak out against this. But our teens also have an important role to play in the advocacy process. Within their schools, teens can talk with the principal or the food service director about offering some healthier food items in the school vending machines. Teens can advocate for change by boycotting products that utilize sexist or weight-loss advertising strategies. They can take things a step further by writing letters to companies, either praising or criticizing the messages they offer, and have their friends sign the letters. Some of the websites previously mentioned offer advice on how best to write these letters. If teens go to the local media with their concerns, they may even be interviewed by the local newspaper or cable TV station. These actions can be effective in turning things around and using the media to advance their cause.

Through these types of empowering activities, girls learn that they don't have to be passive recipients of media messages. Letters written by one Girl Scout troop involved in Free to Be Me were posted on the National Eating Disorders Association media watchdog website; an example is shown in the box on the facing page. The girls turned things around and used the media to get out the messages they believed were important. See the National Eating Disorders Association website (*www.nationaleatingdisorders.org*) for a description of the media watchdog program, the Go Girls program (an excellent media awareness and advocacy program for high school teens), and many other initiatives related to the prevention and treatment of eating disorders.

Do We Have the Power to Make Change Happen?

The Free to Be Me program showed that, at the very least, we can elicit change in the media-related attitudes and behaviors of our kids:

• Following the program, girls were less likely to internalize the thin body ideal portrayed in the media.

• The girls were more likely to believe in their ability to impact weight-related social norms, being more likely to agree with statements such as "I can do something about the types of advertisements shown on TV and in maga-

> Dear Cover Girl,
>
> We are writing because we don't like the advertisements in the October, 1998 issue of YM (*Young and Modern*). All of the people in the ads are skinny and beautiful. Most people aren't really like that. Your ads give girls a negative outlook about their looks since most girls don't look like the ones in your ads. The ads seem to give the message that you have to be skinny to want to wear makeup and look nice—or that if you do wear Cover Girl makeup, then you will become skinny and beautiful.
>
> Please use normal people in your ads, people with all types of body shapes. You don't have to be real thin to want to wear makeup and to want to look nice.
>
> Junior Girl Scouts

zines" and "If someone teased one of my friends about her body size, I would stand up for her and try to be supportive."

- Girls were also more likely to report reading *New Moon* and were less likely to report reading *Seventeen*.

- Troop leaders reported that slightly overweight girls seemed to blossom during the program and "became more a part of the group" than they'd ever been.

- Parents reported that their daughters were pointing out negative messages on billboards and expressing the opinion that the billboards should be taken down, had stopped making negative comments about their bodies, and were beginning to accept their natural body shapes.

We also saw that six sessions are not enough to combat the barrage of media and other negative social influences to which our children are exposed on a daily basis and to impact more ingrained attitudes toward body image and harder-to-change dieting behaviors. An important conclusion that we drew from this study was that parental input and involvement are crucial to change. This program worked so well partly because parents of Girl Scouts tend to be quite involved in their daughters' lives. They volunteer as troop leaders, come to performances given by the girls, and take an interest in their daughters' development. But to bring about meaningful change, parents need to intervene within their homes on an ongoing basis.

In future programs of this type, we hope to involve parents even more by getting them to talk to their daughters about fat talk among peers, weight stigmatization, the media, and other factors influencing body image and dieting behaviors, and making changes within their homes to support positive change. In the meantime, you can adopt some of the activities that we used in Free to Be Me, as described in this chapter. (Also see Chapter 14 for information on how to protect an overweight teen from stigmatization.) You can do a lot to protect your daughter or son from the worst of the media messages and other negative social pressures. And if enough of us make the effort, we may just have an effect on the media themselves and the social environments that surround our teens and our families.

THINKING BIG: MAKING SOCIAL CHANGE HAPPEN

It can feel overwhelming to think about trying to change the social environments that surround our children so that there will be less fat talk, weight stigmatization, and negative media. But Dr. Michael Levine, a world-renowned expert in the prevention of eating disorders, urges us to think back to other major social changes. Thanks to Mothers Against Drunk Driving (MADD), we have changed our views on getting behind the wheel after a drink or two. Social norms in regard to tobacco use have changed drastically over the past 20 years. Women's sports have grown enormously. And look at the civil rights movement. Think big and take small steps toward making a difference ... talk to your teen's peers about dieting norms; talk with your child's coach if weightist remarks are made; write a protest letter to a magazine that includes inappropriate messages; and don't buy the supersize burgers. Through big thoughts and small steps, we can have an impact and make our world one that discourages weight stigmatization and makes it easier for our children to engage in healthier lifestyle behaviors.

Physical Activity

A Big Part of the Answer . . . in Moderation

There's no doubt that physical activity has a lot going for it. Consider Brandy; she shuffles into the house as if she's on her last legs. When her father, Devon, asks her what's wrong, Brandy says with a big yawn, "I'm so, like, *exhausted*."

"What have you been up to?" asks Devon.

"I've been at the mall *all* day."

"Oh, so you did a lot of walking?"

"What? Oh . . . no. We mostly sat around in the courtyard. Everybody was on their cell phones talking to Kate—you know, she and Kafi broke up and she's really upset. We did walk over to the Ice Cream Palace for a sundae later, but, you know, it was just a long day."

Oh.

Now, here's the same girl, walking into the same house, the next day, this time after softball practice:

"*Hey*, Dad, how's it goin'?"

"Great, honey. Looks like *you* had a good day . . . "

Brandy, doing a little dance on her way to the kitchen: "It was awesome. I rocked at practice today. Hey, you wanna play some tennis later?"

You can't see them, but I bet you can imagine them: Brandy no. 1 looks tired, pale, and bored and seems almost unable to move. Brandy no. 2 is glowing, energetic, and ready to play some more.

The two faces of Brandy illustrate just a few of the obvious short-term benefits of physical activity; there are so many others, both short and long term. But is physical activity the panacea for all weight-related problems? And if it is, how do we get teenagers to put it at the center of their lifelong self-care routine?

According to one teen we interviewed, the alternatives—going to the mall or seeing a movie—have a lot going for them, whereas getting sweaty and getting tired are "not, honestly, much fun to some people." Then there's the time factor. Another teenager reeled off a list of obligations that kept her at school 10 to 12 hours a day, took up all day Saturday, and had forced her to quit the soccer team. Maybe we're expecting too much of our teens when we ask them to make physical activity a daily habit.

If we are, it's for good reason: *The percentage of overweight children and teens has tripled over the last 25 years or so,* from about 5% in the early 1970s to 15% in 2000. Over roughly the same time period, walking and bicycling dropped 40% in kids ages 5–15. What are they doing instead? Well, one-third of children and teens today watch TV for more than three hours a day and nearly one-fifth (17%) for more than five hours a day. In 2001 more than a third of our high school girls and about a quarter of the boys were found to have insufficient levels of physical activity.

This fact is particularly disturbing when you realize that what's considered sufficient is probably less than what we parents did for fun without any urging by adults when we were kids: being involved in moderate physical activities for about an hour each day, or nearly every day, and in moderate-to-vigorous levels of exertion three or more times a week for at least 20 minutes.

Technological advances, an abundance of cars, and kids being old enough to get their driver's licenses probably account for a lot of the inactivity of teenagers today, but I bet you haven't really thought about how much less active teenagers are than children. I know I hadn't guessed at the disparity until I read the research. In one study, participation in regular physical activity was reported by 69% of adolescents ages 12–13, but by only 38% of those ages 18–21.

The decline in physical activity is particularly steep for girls. In a 10-year longitudinal study by Dr. Sue Kim and her colleagues, in which more than 2,000 girls were followed from ages 8 to 18, physical activity decreased by 83%, with much larger decreases among the black girls than among the white girls. I've seen this change right before my eyes at my children's middle school, where the boys keep on playing physically active games during recess

PHYSICAL ACTIVITY: WHY THE GENDER GAP?

As teens get older, the gender gap in levels of physical activity gets bigger. Research is exploring what's causing this gap and what might help prevent the large decline in activity in teenage girls. An interview study with African American and Latino middle school girls revealed the following barriers:

1. Many girls struggle with *coed physical education* classes in school and feel they get less attention from the teachers than the boys, are excluded from activities by the boys, and just feel uncomfortable doing certain activities around boys.
2. Girls have *concerns about their appearance* while exercising (for example, hair, sweating, body shape and size, and makeup), particularly around boys.
3. Many of the girls were enthusiastic and interested in physical activity but were frustrated by *inadequate opportunities* to participate.

They also talked about things that help them get moving, such as fun activities (for example, dance or aerobics), social support, and knowing about the positive effects of being active on body image and health. *Social support from family and friends for involvement in fun physical activities is key for increasing physical activity in girls as they approach adolescence.*

but the girls tend to stay inside or walk around a bit outside and talk with each other. A major focus within the public health field has been how to prevent the decline in physical activity among middle school girls. It can and should be a focus for you too.

Let's take a closer look at what our kids are missing out on.

Physical Activity: Why It's Worth the Time and Effort

You know the spiel: Physical activity plays an important role in preventing some of the major health problems of the 21st century, including heart disease and osteoporosis. But are you aware of all the emotional and mental benefits that accrue specifically to teenagers by staying active? The short-term benefits include looking better, feeling better, having a better body image, feeling less stressed, and meeting friends. The details are listed in the following box.

PHYSICAL ACTIVITY CAN HELP TEENS ...

Look better and do more things:

- Helps with weight control, builds lean muscles, and reduces fat.
- May help regulate appetite to eat according to the body's needs.
- Can improve appearance.
- Improves posture.
- Increases muscle strength, flexibility, and aerobic fitness

Feel better in mind and spirit:

- Helps to cope with stress in a healthy way.
- Leads to less tobacco, alcohol, and drug use.
- Reduces feelings of depression and anxiety.
- Increases ability to concentrate and succeed in school.
- Can lead to improved sleep patterns.
- Promotes a feeling of confidence and positive self-esteem.
- Leads to an improved body image.
- Provides opportunities for meeting friends with similar values and interests.
- It's fun!

Be healthier in the long run:

- Helps build and maintain healthy bones.
- Lowers high cholesterol.
- Lowers high blood pressure.
- Decreases risk for heart disease.
- Decreases risk for certain cancers.
- Makes life longer and better!

Any sensible weight management intervention will include physical activity. In fact, for many, it's the focus. That's because as far as scientists know, changing physical activity habits poses less danger of causing a different problem while trying to solve a weight problem than dieting does. Psychologically, deciding to engage in physical activity also feels like a different kind of choice than going on a diet: The former means doing more for yourself and taking better care of yourself, while the latter can lead to feelings of deprivation. Furthermore, *physical activity has been shown to help in weight maintenance and in the prevention of regaining weight after losing it*. Anyone who has ever lost weight knows that it's easier to lose weight than to keep it off; physical activity can help.

Talk about the benefits of physical activity for weight loss and, more important, for the prevention of weight gain. But be sure to also talk about how physical activity can help with stress management, improvement of appearance and body image, meeting new friends and having fun with old ones, and overall health promotion and disease prevention. By focusing on the many benefits of physical activity, you have an opportunity to encourage a behavior with positive implications for weight management, without overemphasizing weight issues.

Why Physical Activity Is No Cure-All

The benefits are undeniable, but is that all there is to the story on physical activity?

EXERCISING ISN'T A MAGIC PILL FOR LOSING WEIGHT

I'm concerned that physical activity is being pushed as the answer to all our problems. I think certain food manufacturers are trying to "get off the hook" by claiming it's not their products but the decline in physical activity that's responsible for obesity. Does anyone else see the irony of Coke and McDonald's sponsoring programs aimed at increasing physical activity? (Just check out their websites if you don't believe they're doing this.)

Judging by the ads for fitness equipment, anyone who works out can expect to become superlean and ripped. But, of course, it's not that simple. Neither, for that matter, is losing weight by exercising. Moderate physical activity cannot, on its own, counteract the impact of large portions of foods high in fats and sugars. Even when combined with healthier diets, it's not going to produce losses of 30-pounds-in-30-days proportions. But teenagers will be teenagers. They want satisfaction, and they want it fast. I've known kids who were justifiably proud of going from no activity to a half-hour walk a day but then gave up on it when it didn't produce any weight loss. One teenager I know went to her mother frustrated and dejected and demanding to know why she hadn't gotten any skinnier—after all, for a whole week she'd been working out every day and eating less.

Physical Activity

what you can do
HELP YOUR TEENS GET REAL
ABOUT EXPECTATIONS

Teens need to get a realistic perspective on what they can expect from physical activity in terms of weight control. Although I don't like to focus on calories too much, you might point out to your kids that the calories burned off by 30 minutes of running will easily be replaced by one large soda pop and a bag of potato chips. They should also know that with exercise come changes in body composition due to increased lean body mass, which actually can weigh more than fat but is healthier, looks better, and burns more calories. So, changes may not show up on the scale but will be evident in the way your son or daughter looks and feels.

THERE'S SUCH A THING AS TOO MUCH OF A GOOD THING

When I recently gave a talk in Sydney, Australia, I quoted a girl who happily reported starting to go to the gym several times a week. A member of the audience challenged my presenting this statement as positive, saying that the eating disorders that brought many teenagers to her treatment center often started with "going to the gym." To her, proud announcements about going to the gym regularly were a red flag for potential eating disorders.

So, when we encourage teenagers to exercise more, we need to realize that some teens will take the message too far. Where does that leave us? The Sydney seminar came up with a solution that made sense: When you encourage your son or daughter to be physically active, put the focus on enjoyment. Appropriate messages might be "Find activities that you like to do! Try new activities." "Enjoy the way your body feels when it's active. Have fun!" It's not much different from eating: When you stop enjoying your food because you're satiated, you should stop eating. If exercise isn't largely enjoyable, something is wrong, and it may be that you're doing it to excess. Kids with anorexia nervosa or anorexia athletica no longer experience a sense of enjoyment in physical activity, but rather a compulsion to do more.

We need to avoid pushing our kids too hard to be active or to stick with a sport against their will. This can be hard to do if we've invested a lot in our teens' progress and see that they have real ability. It can be particularly hard if a possible college acceptance or scholarship is riding on such a talent. But the stakes associated with pushing a kid too far are just too high.

Even when our children are not star athletes, we need to be getting the message across that physical activity should be fun . . . at least most of the time. Take a look at how you talk. Compare the following two statements that could be made after a long nature hike:

- "It was so great to go hiking today; the weather was perfect, the scenery was beautiful, and I just loved getting some exercise."
- "That was a great hike today. I really got my heart rate up there . . . although I could have pushed myself a bit more."

Or take this example: Just as I finished writing the last sentence, my son called me after a high school tennis match. I asked how it went and he replied, "It sucked. I lost." I waited a moment and then he said, "But it was cool." So I replied, "As long as you had fun. That's the main thing."

We also need to be aware of when things may be going a bit too far for our kids. Signs indicating that a teen's physical activity is going beyond the enjoyment phase include behaviors such as getting up to run when feeling sick or in the worst of weather (although here in Minnesota that seems to be the norm for many people I know); giving up fun activities such as sleep-overs because they'll cut into exercise time, and displaying signs of distress when his or her exercise routine is interrupted. It can be hard to distinguish between what is normal and what is too much if your teen is involved in a highly competitive activity. In fact, Drs. Ron Thompson and Roberta Sherman, experts in the study of eating disorders among athletes, have found that some eating disorder symptoms, such as weight loss and excessive exercise, may be valued within the sports world, and that some characteristics common to people with anorexia are just extreme counterparts of qualities prized by athletes—such as perfectionism (common in anorexia), as compared with the pursuit of excellence (characteristic of athletes).

OVEREMPHASIZING EXERCISE CAN LEAD TO OVEREMPHASIZING MUSCLE MASS AND USING STEROIDS

For some teens, particularly boys, body dissatisfaction focuses on muscle mass. Just as we impress on our children that beauty comes in different sizes, we need to send the message that physical fitness can occur with different sizes and shapes. Unfortunately, the popularity of weightlifting gyms has increased the perception that excessive bodybuilding is desirable. I don't know about you, but I am amazed at the inordinate amounts of time teenage boys and young men spend weightlifting at a gym. In addition, high school sports have become so competitive that many boys feel they need an edge beyond what they get from natural talent and lots of practice in their sport. As a result, many teens today are experimenting with different kinds of supplements, such as weight-gain powders and protein drinks. Of greater concern, however, is the use of anabolic steroids to enhance muscle growth.

Use of anabolic steroids during adolescence can interfere with bone growth; damage internal organs such as the heart or liver; cause sterility; lead to feminization in boys, such as breast development; and lead to masculinization in girls, such as the development of facial hair. Teens who are considering using steroids to promote muscle development must be made aware of these consequences.

In Project EAT, 5% of the boys and 3% of the girls reported using anabolic steroids to gain muscle in the past year. Although these numbers may not seem very high, they are of great concern in light of the potential consequences associated with the use of steroids. And other reports show that steroid use is on the rise; the Monitoring the Future Survey, an ongoing national study of more than 40,000 8th, 10th, and 12th graders, has found that while use of most illegal drugs has been leveling off or decreasing, anabolic steroid use is increasing in teenage boys. Furthermore, in 2002 the perceived risk of using steroids was lower than it had ever been before. Teens in Project EAT who were using steroids tended to be more preoccupied with their weight and body shape. They also tended to have less knowledge about nutrition and health, suggesting a need for discussing these issues at home and at school to avoid common misconceptions. Teens who don't know the basics about nutrition and health may be more vulnerable to media messages promoting all kinds of bodybuilding substances. Teens need to know that protein powders and steroids are not appropriate substitutes for proper nutrition and physical activity. Our teens need to have the skills to be able to distinguish fact from fiction in regard to messages about health and fitness.

---

what you can do
HELP YOUR SON UNDERSTAND THE DANGERS OF USING BODYBUILDING SUBSTANCES

➡Reinforce the notion that people, and particularly teens, have all different shapes and sizes. Assure your teenagers that they are normal.

➡If you have a teenage boy who is a late developer, remind him again and again that he will grow to become taller and more muscular.

➡Discuss the dangers of supplements, muscle enhancers, and steroids. Tell your teens to beware of anything that promises too much.

→Stress that food is the best source of nutrients, since it provides a balance of whatever you need. Plus, there is still so much that supplement developers don't know ... so you are better off getting whatever you need naturally from a balanced diet.

→Let your teens know that a person's body can use only so much protein. Above and beyond what is needed will not turn into extra muscle but will be excreted in urine. The vast majority of teens get more than enough protein.

→Talk about the advertising techniques used to sell products. Just as models in the media may be computer-modified to make them look thinner, pictures may be touched up to enhance muscles (see Chapter 4).

→Get your teen a book on the topic. A comprehensive book, designed as a college textbook, is *Nutrition for Health, Fitness, and Sport* by Melvin Williams (see Resources).

→Make an appointment with your primary health care provider. Let your doctor know about your concerns prior to the meeting. Your teen may be more likely to listen to an expert on the topic than to a parent.

→Ask your son and his friends if they really think extreme bodybuilders are healthy. If girls are around, get their opinions. Boys may be surprised to hear that the girls think some of these guys are "just gross."

→As always, check out your own behaviors and your spouse's. What kinds of messages are you giving your teens about an ideal body shape, an appropriate amount of time to be spending weightlifting, and the use of supplements.

SOME SPORTS EMPHASIZE WEIGHT AND BODY SHAPE

Do you have a teen involved in wrestling, boxing, figure skating, dance, gymnastics, or other sports that emphasize body weight and shape? Are you worried about your child feeling pressured to conform to a very thin body shape? Do you wonder whether your daughter's self-esteem will be affected if she takes a shot at the elite levels of her sport but doesn't excel? As the mother of a daughter who likes to dance and do gymnastics, and as a professional who hears the tip-of-the-iceberg horror stories, I've had questions like these. So I reviewed the research that had been done in this area, and our research team did some investigation of its own.

Research shows that teens participating in weight-related sports are at greater risk for disordered eating practices than others. This is particularly true for those participating at the elite level. But we've also found that girls participating in weight-related sports were at decreased risk for other unhealthy behaviors, such as tobacco and marijuana use. So you may need to weigh the pros and the cons, taking into account your own child's vulnerability (refer to the worksheet you filled out in Chapter 2).

In our research, we found that only certain girls participating in weight-related sports were at higher risk for disordered eating behaviors. The more vulnerable girls were those who engaged in other unhealthy behaviors, including the use of tobacco, alcohol, marijuana, and other drugs; those who had experienced some type of physical or sexual abuse; those displaying depressive symptoms; and girls who reported difficulties in family relationships (for example, found it hard to talk to their parents). Preexisting weight-related concerns and problematic eating behaviors, as well as personality factors, should also be taken into account. A kid with perfectionist tendencies may be affected negatively, whereas a well-adjusted kid who knows how to roll with the punches and generally feels good about herself is probably at low risk. Besides assessing the child's personal vulnerabilities, you'll want to investigate the program thoroughly.

what you can do
INVESTIGATE THE WEIGHT-RELATED ATTITUDES OF ANY SPORTS PROGRAM

What are the demands of the program and the attitudes of the instructors regarding body weight? Do participants seem pressured to conform to a specific body shape and size? Or is there acceptance of a variety of shapes and sizes? Are there any discussions about dieting or healthy eating at the program? What do the instructors do if they suspect that a participant might be at risk for an eating disorder? When do they get in touch with parents? Do they work with a dietitian?

Ask these questions, but also make your own observations. Diversity, or a lack thereof, in the body shapes and sizes of the instructors and the students can tell you a lot!

what you can do
MAKE YOUR EXPECTATIONS CLEAR TO YOUR TEENAGERS WHEN THEY START PARTICIPATING IN A WEIGHT-RELATED SPORT

Tell your teens that you're concerned about any possible pressure to conform to a particular body shape, and say you think they look great as they are; tell them that health comes first, and that if you see them restricting their dietary intake or engaging in excessive exercise, you won't let them continue to participate. Also take another look at your own weight concerns and behaviors to make sure you and your spouse are being appropriate role models for your teens. It's important to filter out excessive and unhealthy pressures regarding weight and to avoid reinforcing those messages via your own behaviors. Furthermore, a bit more care should be taken to have family meals on a regular basis, to touch base with your teens, talk about how things are going, and see that they're getting a healthy diet. If problems do emerge, address them immediately with your teen, the program instructor, and a health care provider. *Signs indicating that there may be a problem include any of the following: weight loss, loss of menstrual cycles, excessive exercise, use of exercise to burn off calories after eating a larger-than-normal amount of food, unhealthy dieting behaviors, and changes in normal tasks of adolescent development such as withdrawing from socializing or decreased academic achievement.*

How to Encourage Your Teen to Get More Active (without Going Overboard)

In total, the research certainly shows that physical activity is important for physical and mental health. Although some teens go overboard, most teens aren't active enough. Teenagers should engage in moderate physical activity pretty much every day and in more vigorous activity at least 20 minutes a day three times a week. More than that is fine too—within limits. How do you make that happen?

Jerome's mother would like to see her son be a bit more physically active. He comes home from school, and his activity seems to consist of walking from the couch facing the television, to his desk for homework and computer use, to the fridge for a snack. When she raises her concerns about his low level of physical activity, he says he just doesn't have time because of his demanding academic schedule. Furthermore, he just can't seem to get motivated to be active; he can't think of any activities that he really enjoys doing, his friends aren't involved in sports and he doesn't want to go at it alone, and he isn't good enough to go out for any high school sports anyhow. Jerome's mom just isn't sure what to say or do to help him out.

My research team decided that to be able to offer solutions to problems like this family's, we really had to get a firmer idea of the obstacles to getting appropriate exercise that teenagers experience. So in individual interviews we asked teenagers to tell us what makes it hard for them to be physically active and what helps them to be more active. Using survey data, we examined associations between the level of physical activity and a range of personal and socioenvironmental factors. The information we got helped me crystallize a few effective strategies.

STRATEGIES FOR HELPING YOUR TEEN BE MORE PHYSICALLY ACTIVE

Strategy 1: To Get Around the "I'm Too Busy" Obstacle, Help Your Teens Replace Sedentary Time with Active Time

Research has shown that teens are either too busy to squeeze in physical activity or think they're too busy. It's true that many teens have very busy schedules, but it's also true that most of the kids we talked to reported spending lots of time— usually more than planned—surfing the net or watching TV. In the same research study, in which time constraints emerged as the strongest obstacle to physical activity, teenage girls reported that they watched an average of nearly three hours of television a *day*, but spent only three hours a *week* in moderate to vigorous physical activity! So it may be worthwhile for Jerome's mother to help him out with some time management skills, to help him realize how he currently spends his time and how he could fit in some physical activity.

Some of the teens we interviewed talked about how having a schedule would help them stay physically active. In one of our programs, the teens tracked their level of inactivity over a three-day period using the form on the facing page. Then they thought about how they could reduce their sedentary time and substitute physical activities for some of that time. If you can get your teens to write down how much time they spend in the activities listed on the form, and then think about how to reduce that time—great! If not, a discussion with your teens about how much time gets eaten up with activities such as watching television can be useful. Don't come down on them; the aim should be to get them to realize how they spend their time as a first step toward change. You may find it helpful to focus on yourself and discuss how things like television and e-mail eat up your time and how you're trying to deal with this situation. Some other ideas for overcoming the obstacle of just not having enough time for physical activity are shown in the box on page 94.

TRACKING INACTIVITY

To help you assess the amount of time you spend being inactive, complete this worksheet for three days (two weekdays and one weekend day).

Day 1	Minutes/Hours
Watching TV	_____
Computer time	_____
Playing video games	_____
Reading/homework	_____
Talking on the phone	_____
Listening to music (not moving)	_____
Sitting or lying around	_____
Other: _____	_____

Day 2	Minutes/Hours
Watching TV	_____
Computer time	_____
Playing video games	_____
Reading/homework	_____
Talking on the phone	_____
Listening to music (not moving)	_____
Sitting or lying around	_____
Other: _____	_____

Day 3	Minutes/Hours
Watching TV	_____
Computer time	_____
Playing video games	_____
Reading/homework	_____
Talking on the phone	_____
Listening to music (not moving)	_____
Sitting or lying around	_____
Other: _____	_____

Physical Activity

IS YOUR TEEN "TOO BUSY" FOR PHYSICAL ACTIVITY?

Share These Time-Saving Ideas with your Teen ...

- Set a maximum time for daily TV watching or going on-line. If that doesn't work, set a timer to remind you that an hour has just passed.

- Don't have a television in your room—you will spend more time watching it!

- Keep a record of how much time you actually spend in sedentary activities—you may be surprised!

- Do some type of physical activity while watching TV or talking on the phone: keep a pair of weights, a stretch band, and a big resistance ball nearby. Or walk on a treadmill while watching your favorite show.

- Aim to substitute 30 minutes of sedentary behavior with 30 minutes of active time each day. Just cut out one TV show and go for a short walk.

- Try to put more action in your normal daily activities such as taking the stairs instead of the elevator or biking to your friend's house instead of getting a ride.

- Jump rope for three minutes before you take a shower.

- Do five minutes of stretching when you get up in the morning.

- Integrate physical activity into your social life: When getting together with friends, suggest activities such as roller-blading, swimming, or biking.

- No time after school? Sign up for an elective physical education class at your school.

- Next time your family is talking about a family vacation, suggest making it an active one.

- After school, before homework, take an activity break instead of a television break. Your body and mind will benefit. Stick in an aerobics video instead of another movie and move to it.

- Get a summer job that involves some type of moving around, such as refereeing soccer games, being an assistant coach, teaching swimming, or working at a summer camp. You'll get great experience, make some money, and be active.

- Babysitting? Take the kids for a bike ride, put on a CD and dance with them, bring along an aerobics video and do the moves together, or offer to take the kids roller-blading.

Strategy 2: Support Your Teen's Efforts to Get Active

In our research, we found that teens who felt they received support for physical activity from their parents, peers, and teachers were more physically active. Make sure your teen knows that you think physical activity deserves a spot every day just like academics and other activities—and that it's worth the hour of time even if that means cutting into time allotted for hitting the book or hanging with friends. Here are some other ideas:

- Help your adolescent find an exercise partner—maybe you. Most of the teens we interviewed said an exercise partner would help keep them motivated to be physically active by preventing boredom and making the time pass faster.
- Talk about the importance of physical activity and its many benefits.
- Model a physically active lifestyle. Remember that teens are most likely to emulate your physically active lifestyle if they see you being active.
- Provide or arrange for transportation to sporting events, classes, or other opportunities for physical activity.
- Help out with the "behind the scenes" work, such as filling out forms, looking for suitable activities, and paying the registration fees.
- Try to facilitate friendships with other physically active teenagers.
- Plan for active family time (after dinner, on weekends, or on a vacation). Do this instead of watching TV or going to a movie.
- Encourage your teens to participate in community and school sports.
- Go watch them participate!

Jerome's mother might want to take a look at their home atmosphere: Is physical activity the norm in the house? If not, what could be changed? Perhaps the pattern of television use needs to be changed, with hours of use more restricted. She could try to enlist Jerome's help in getting her to be active; perhaps they could buy two pedometers, put together a walking plan, and try to go a bit farther each evening. This would also provide them with an opportunity to talk. In planning for their next family vacation, they could think of active options that might include biking, hiking, or swimming. If you're concerned about your own teen's level of physical activity, take a look at your home environment, ask yourself whether it is one that supports physical activity, and if not, what you could work on to change it.

what you can do
GET THEM TO HELP *YOU* STAY ACTIVE

Hector Sztainer, a physical education teacher (and my husband), strongly suggests getting your teens to help you be more active. Tell your teens that you need some social support, and get them to go for a walk or a bike ride with you. This has the added benefit of providing a chance for schmoozing with your teens that might not happen otherwise.

Strategy 3: Be Sensitive to Your Teen's Insecurities

I can't emphasize enough how important it is to be sensitive to the fact that many teenagers who are not already active are very self-conscious about exercising. If they're overweight, they may fear they'll be teased about how they look while exercising—and this fear may be based on experience. Not surprisingly, a study on more than 500 5th to 8th graders found that children who were criticized about their weight during physical activity enjoyed such activity significantly less than their peers. If children have never been athletic, they may think someone will make fun of their lack of skill. Being made to feel bad about their appearance or performance level can have devastating effects on a teenager's self-esteem and body image.

So, what *can* you do or say to urge your teenager to be more active while remaining sensitive to his or her legitimate concerns?

NEW MOVES: A NEW APPROACH FOR INCREASING PHYSICAL ACTIVITY IN SEDENTARY GIRLS

We ran an alternative, supportive physical education program called New Moves for high school girls who were either overweight or at risk for becoming overweight as a result of sedentary lifestyles. The girls set goals for gradual changes in physical activity according to their current levels. They were exposed to a range of different types of activities that could be done at different body shapes and sizes, such as aerobic dance, yoga, kickboxing, hiking, snowshoeing, and weight lifting. Afterward, the girls said that engaging in physical activity in a noncompetitive, supportive atmosphere improved their confidence in their ability to get moving, overall self-esteem, and body image. They stressed the fact that the program had not focused on trying to get them to lose weight. They said it made them understand that, because there's no such thing as physical perfection, "you can feel good for who you are and how you look." One girl said she used to hate her body—"But now I like it," she reported.

- Do whatever you can to help your teen find an environment in which she will feel comfortable being active. Is there a *place* in your community that is more likely to attract kids of different sizes? The YWCA may be better than your local fitness club. Are there *instructors* of different shapes, sizes, or ethnicities? Your teen may feel more comfortable with someone who looks like her. Are there *activities* in which size is less important? Yoga, pilates, self-defense, weightlifting, water aerobics, volleyball, and certain types of dance may work well for your teen regardless of her size. Is there a *supportive atmosphere* that encourages gradual change and provides positive reinforcement? The New Moves program worked well because it included kids of all sizes, guest instructors from different backgrounds, a range of activities in which size didn't get in the way of things, and a very supportive environment. Teens need a setting in which they can feel comfortable. So if your teen hates getting all sweaty and out of breath, suggest options such as swimming, dance, yoga, and weight lifting. If your teen isn't good enough to make a school team, look for alternatives such as jazz, hip hop, or aerobics classes at a local community center. And outdoor activities such as biking, hiking, canoeing, or skiing, either in a club or with some friends, tend to make us feel good about what we are able to do with our bodies . . . without having to worry about how we look.

- If your teen expresses concerns about what others will think when they see him running the mile, doing a cartwheel, or lifting weights, don't just exhort your teen to "get out there and do it." Instead, talk openly with your teen about how he's feeling and what types of options might work for him.

- Take a look at what you are modeling. Are you hesitant to put on shorts, go swimming, or go to the gym because of how you look (if your body is less than perfect). Try taking a new approach. Do these things anyway and say something like "I may not be the most coordinated person in the class, but I feel so proud of myself for showing up and doing what I can."

- Reframe sentences such as "I feel so fat and out of shape" to "I feel so good about my body after I push myself a bit" or "I used to be able to walk for only five minutes, and now I'm up to a half-hour."

- When you're watching others compete, dance, or participate in a show, look for opportunities to make comments such as "I think it's great that kids of all shapes and sizes are competing." Avoid comments like "She'd look more graceful if she were a bit thinner."

- Acknowledge your teen's difficulties and brainstorm coping strategies. "It's hard to put on a swimsuit when you think everyone is going to be talking behind your back. Some kids might laugh . . . but others might admire your boldness. What are some things you can do if someone makes a rude remark? How might you preempt an attack?"

• Don't force, or even push, your teen to do activities in which she knows she won't feel comfortable. Instead, talk about alternatives that would work for her. "All of us have to decide what works for us . . . what are some activities you would feel comfortable doing?"

• Think about yourself and the times when being physically active made you feel better about yourself and your body. What were you doing? Who was with you? What kinds of comments did others make that were supportive? What were you saying to yourself? Incorporate the kinds of experiences that you've found helpful into your comments and actions with your own teens.

Strategy 4: Make It Fun!

Hector Sztainer, the physical education instructor and spouse whom I mentioned earlier, is a huge proponent of helping teens find physical activities that work for them. For many teens, the social (or schmoozing) aspects of being involved in sports can be a big attraction and can be used to help encourage your teens to get involved. But for some teens, individualized activities, in which the social component is rather minimal, may be more suitable. We're more likely to be physically active if we like what we're doing. But sometimes when we think about physical activity we start thinking in terms of "shoulds" instead of "wants." We might say things like "I should start working out." It would be so much better if we could see things more positively and say things like "I can't wait to play tennis after work."

One of the high school girls who participated in the New Moves program listed a whole slew of activities that she liked to do, probably more than she would have predicted before participating in the program—from snowshoeing to jumping rope, walking, weight lifting, and horseback riding—all of which she described as "just fun." "When I do them I don't even realize that they're working out stuff," she said. Your teens may need some help in finding activities that work best for them. Does your daughter like music? Maybe she'd enjoy a dance class or club—like one of the girls we interviewed, who joined the school's salsa club with a friend and had a great time. Another said that she just loved walking and lost weight in summer because the weather was good enough to walk everywhere, but she even walked a lot during the winter at indoor malls. If your teenager can't come up with any ideas, you need to help her think outside the box a bit. Show her the chart here.

99 IDEAS FOR GETTING ACTIVE

Throw a ball

Snowshoe for fun

Stretch while watching TV

Lift weights by the TV

Go on a canoe trip

Shoot some hoops

Turn on music and dance

Frisbee golf

Frisbee

Climb a mountain

Play hopscotch

Hop on a treadmill

Try a fancy exercise machine

Aerobic dance

Play in the snow

Swim laps

Dive off a board

Walk after dinner

Badminton

Ethnic dancing

Swing dancing

Hip-hop

Take a study break

Racquetball

Weight lifting at a gym

Walk around a mall

Walk to your locker between classes

Weed your garden

Try playing squash

Hop on a horse

Walk with a pedometer

Try downhill skiing

Try martial arts

Go skateboarding

Try snowboarding

Roller-blade

Roller-skate at a rink

Go down a water slide

Jump rope for 2 minutes

Try skipping for fun

Shovel your driveway

Go up and down your stairs

Play tennis

Golf, anyone?

Basketball pickup game

Soccer game

Go sledding

Hula hoop for 2 minutes

Volleyball at the beach

Floor hockey

Ice hockey

Walk with a friend

Walk with your phone

Do sit-ups for 3 minutes

Get on a resistance ball

How about rugby?

Mow your lawn

Mow your neighbor's lawn

Jump rope backwards

Plant a vegetable garden

Try jogging

Take a jazz class

Pilates

Yoga

Play on a playground

Train for a marathon

Go for a bike ride

Do 10 jumping jacks

Stretch by the computer

Ice skating

Gymnastics

How about lacrosse?

Try kickboxing

Cross-country skiing

Circuit training

Rowboating

Water skiing

Try water aerobics

Go dancing with friends

Ultimate Frisbee

Hike in nature

Walk around a lake

Play with children

Do yoga sun salutations

Try juggling

Do five push-ups

Get on a scooter

Do a cartwheel

Walk your dog

Walk your cat???

Strategy 5: Help Your Teens Think about Gradual Changes So They Don't Get Discouraged and Lose Self-Confidence

Success builds on prior successes, so starting slowly is recommended for promoting self-confidence. If your son hasn't been physically active and now he's decided he'll start running every evening for an hour, he may easily get discouraged. You could suggest reasonable goals, maybe starting with a 20-minute walk three times a week, five minutes of stretching every morning, or going to the pool once a week.

Strategy 6: Emphasize Balance

Yes, physical activity is a big part of the solution to weight-related problems. But it's not the entire answer, and there can be too much of a good thing. In encouraging your teenagers to get more active, remember to emphasize balance. When your son is so pumped up from working out every afternoon that he wants to go out for a run right after dinner too, remind him that life is more than exercise and suggest he read a book instead. When your daughter who works at a strenuous lifeguard job announces she's going to the health club first thing on the morning of her day off, ask why and tell her she deserves her time off to have some fun.

Meanwhile, strive for a little balance for yourself too. You can't make your teens be physically active. Remember that they are teens and the final decision will be their own. Too much pressure will backfire and may lead to either too little or too much physical activity. In Chapter 7 we look more closely at how to address the question of balance when trying to help our teens.

6

The Great Diet Debate

*D*ieting is so common among teenage girls that the question "Are you on a diet?" may be less meaningful than "Which diet are you on?"
Is anything wrong with this picture? I'll let you be the judge.

The "negatives" of dieting:

- Dieting can lead to feelings of restriction and deprivation, which can lead to binge eating.
- Over time, dieting has been found to lead to weight gain in teens—instead of weight loss.
- "Going on a diet" can be the first step in the chain of events leading to a clinical eating disorder for some teens.
- Teens who engage in unhealthy dieting are at risk of not getting the nutrients their bodies need.
- Kids who diet can have psychological problems too; most notably dieting can lead to depression.

The "positives" of dieting:

-
-
-
-
-

Oh. I guess there is one: Dieting is big business. Lots of money is being made on the sales of diet books, programs, and products. Maybe those who diet are contributing to a healthy economy.

Now, if only going on a diet contributed to a healthy body and mind . . .

I may be overstating the case. The topic of dieting is pretty controversial, in part because different people mean different things by "dieting," but also because dieting is still viewed as the standard treatment for obesity. Yet over the years I've become more and more convinced that dieting is not the way to go. This conclusion is based on my clinical work with adults who have struggled unsuccessfully with dieting for years, and on my research findings, which have revealed an alarmingly high prevalence of dieting among preteens: *One-third of fifth-grade girls in the United States report that they have already been on a diet.* It's also based on many conversations with health care professionals throughout the world and a comprehensive review of the scientific literature, all of which point to the fact that dieting is ineffective and, worse, harmful.

What Do We Mean by "Dieting" or "Going on a Diet"?

I'm sure you haven't given much thought to the kinds of statements listed below when a friend or your teenager utters them. But take the opportunity to look at them more closely now. They reveal a lot about what we mean by *dieting*.

Things people say when they are planning to go on a diet, are on a diet, or have "broken" their diet:

"I'm starting my diet on Monday." (*implied: and it's Saturday, so I can eat whatever I want.*)

"I need to lose 10 pounds quickly. I'll do a crash diet for two weeks and then start eating healthfully." (*The problem: It just doesn't happen like this.*)

"I was so hungry when I got home from school that I just grabbed a bag of chips."

"I had trouble concentrating in my class (or meeting) before lunch because my stomach was growling." (*After skipping breakfast.*)

"Well, I already broke my diet." (*Implied: So it doesn't matter what I eat for the rest of the day.*)

"I'm so upset with myself. I broke my diet with a few spoonfuls of ice cream and then ended up eating nearly a half gallon."

"I don't think I should go to the party on Saturday night; they'll probably have good food, and I just started a new diet and I don't want to blow it."

"I started a new diet two days ago. Now I'm hungrier than ever, because I'm thinking about food all the time."

"I just couldn't resist having a piece of the chocolate cake. I feel as though I have no self-control; I am just so upset with myself."

These are things I heard constantly when I ran weight control groups for adults 20 years ago, when I began my career as a dietitian. In those days, I too believed in the power of diet plans and weekly weigh-ins. But then I started lying in bed at night thinking about comments that my clients made, such as "I was so bad this week" or "I cheated" or "Next week I'll be better and I won't eat any chocolate." It became apparent to me that while I was weighing their bodies, they were weighing their self-worth. Can you see why they eventually made me change my thinking about dieting and how best to achieve long-term weight changes? Can you guess why they led me to working with teenagers, to prevent the problems before they occur? *By its nature,* dieting is doomed to failure, and yet dieters always blame themselves for not achieving the goals they've started the diet to reach. A lot of heartache is left in the wake of a million "failed" diets. Which leads me to my definition of *dieting*:

> **Dieting for weight loss:** An eating plan that includes rigid rules about what to eat, how much, in what combinations, or at what times, that is usually followed for a specified period, for the purpose of weight loss.

Using this definition, examples of dieting would include the following weight loss plans: 1,000 calories per day diet, 1,200 calories per day diet, Atkins diet, Sugar Busters diet, banana and yogurt diet, and the grapefruit diet. Strict rules about eating, also followed for the purpose of weight loss, would be included here as well, such as total elimination of desserts or "extras," no mixing proteins with carbohydrates at meals, or no eating until dinnertime.

I'm sure you can see the two key features in the definition of *dieting* that demonstrate why it's problematic: *strict rules* about eating, followed on a *temporary* basis. Rules about eating often lead to feelings of deprivation, which in turn lead to the breaking of rules. Once rules are broken, the dieter "goes wild" until starting the diet again. How often have you heard someone say something like "Well, I already broke my diet, so why not? I'll start again after the weekend." Furthermore, dieting is typically viewed as a temporary behavior: "I need to go on a diet to lose 10 pounds before my cousin's wedding." It is often viewed as a "project." But for long-term weight change and maintenance, ongoing lifestyle changes that allow for some flexibility are needed.

Why Not Diet?

THE DIET–BINGE CYCLE

It all goes back to Adam and Eve. Eve wanted the apple as soon as eating it became forbidden. This is the problem with dieting. As soon as foods become forbidden, we want them more. And when we eat these forbidden foods and then feel guilty, we often end up eating large quantities because we know they'll soon become forbidden again. In a study I did with teenage girls in Israel, binge eating was three times higher among girls using unhealthy weight control behaviors (45%) than among the other girls (15%).

This diet–binge cycle is depicted in the following diagram. Anyone who has dieted can relate to this vicious circle. Different people respond to feelings

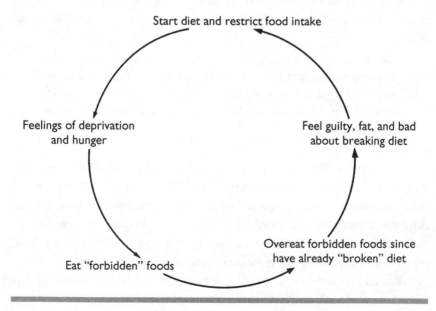

The diet–binge cycle.

of deprivation and hunger with different degrees of overeating, but generally bingeing will be more common among teenagers using unhealthy weight control behaviors, who have low self-esteem or a poor body image, or who tend to overeat to cope with difficult emotional or social situations.

DIETS JUST DON'T WORK—IN FACT, THEY CAN LEAD TO WEIGHT GAIN

If dieting worked, would obesity be on the rise the way it is? The National Eating Disorders Association estimates that 40–50% of American women are trying to lose weight at any point in time. In a national study of youth that we did, 56% of high school girls and 23% of high school boys, plus 36% of girls in late elementary and middle school and 18% of boys of the same age reported dieting behaviors. These figures don't indicate that dieting is causing an increase in obesity, but they certainly do suggest that it isn't doing much to prevent it.

Whether dieting helps people maintain any weight loss they achieve is an ongoing controversy, and the research evidence varies. But I can tell you that the statistic quoted most commonly is that 95% of people who lose weight on diets gain it back. Anecdotal evidence and clinical experience back this up. I can't tell you many times I've heard an overweight adult say, "If only I hadn't started dieting when I was a teenager, I would be much thinner now." Reasons for this pattern are not 100% clear, but may include metabolic disturbances, in which dieting causes a reduction in the resting metabolic rate, and behavioral disturbances, whereby it becomes harder and harder to keep behaving in ways that support weight maintenance.

The most compelling evidence demonstrating that dieting not only doesn't produce lasting weight loss but may also lead to weight gain in teens comes from two studies in which teenagers were followed over a number of years. *In both of these studies, dieters were found to gain weight over time, not lose weight*:

- Dr. Eric Stice and his colleagues studied nearly 700 teenage girls over the 4-year high school period. *Girls who dieted in ninth grade were more than three times as likely to be overweight in twelfth grade, as compared with girls who did not diet in ninth grade.* This was not due to the fact that the dieters started off heavier than the other girls, because the researchers made statistical adjustments for any differences in body weight at the beginning of the study and excluded from the analysis girls who were originally overweight.
- Dr. Alison Field and her colleagues found similar patterns in a study of

15,000 girls and boys, ages 9–14, who were followed for 3 years. They found that teens who dieted were more likely to gain weight than nondieters. *Furthermore, they found that dieters were much more likely to binge than nondieters.* Girls who dieted frequently were twelve times more likely to binge than nondieters. Among boys, frequent dieters were seven times more likely to binge than nondieters. These findings led the study authors to speculate that repeated cycles of overeating, between periods of restrictive dieting, might have been responsible for the increased weight gain among the dieters.

A FIRST STEP TOWARD DISORDERED EATING AND EATING DISORDERS

Many of the mass media reports about anorexia and bulimia that you may have seen have raised an alarm about the connection between dieting and eating disorders, and there's a grain of truth there. Those in the field of eating disorders have been taking a hard look at this question and have found that, on its own, dieting will probably not lead to an eating disorder. However, because of all the spheres of influence described in Chapter 2 and the developmental challenges that make teenagers particularly vulnerable, dieting usually doesn't occur on its own. The facts are these: Most dieters do not progress to more serious disordered eating behaviors or develop an eating disorder. But virtually all of those who are diagnosed with an eating disorder or engage in some form of disordered eating have dieted in the past.

Dieting may lead to disordered eating via a number of paths. For example, teens with low self-worth, who tend to be perfectionists or are achievement oriented, are depressed, or feel the need to gain some control may get satisfaction from losing weight. If this self-satisfaction is reinforced by compliments from others who equate thinness with beauty, the teenager may decide she's onto something and pursue the dieting even more vigorously than at first.

This link was confirmed by a study of 2,000 Australian teenagers conducted by Dr. George Patton and his research team, who classified teens as "severe" or "moderate" dieters according to how strictly they counted calories, reduced their food intake, and skipped meals. The team found that the *chances of developing a partial or full eating disorder within a 12-month period were 1 in 5 for severe dieters, 1 in 40 for moderate dieters, and fewer than 1 in 500 for nondieters.*

The message is clear; dieting behaviors in teenage girls should not be viewed as innocuous. For some teens such behaviors may be the last step in a chain of events, but for others they may be only the first step. Knowing this makes it clear how important it is for us to try to get our teens to avoid them in the first place, or at the very least to keep them healthy, minimal, and monitored.

JUST WHEN IT COUNTS MOST, DIETING CAN REDUCE YOUR CHILD'S NUTRIENT INTAKE

Teens who diet, particularly teenage girls who use unhealthy weight control behaviors, are missing out on some critical nutrients. In Project EAT, cutting down on dairy foods, a typical restriction, left 75% of the girls using unhealthy weight control behaviors consuming less than the recommended amount of calcium. This may not seem like a big deal until you consider the fact that nearly half of a person's skeletal mass is added during adolescence. Those who reach their optimal peak bone mass at this time are ahead of the game when they are adults and their bones start losing calcium as part of the normal aging process.

I'm sure you can just imagine the eye rolling or blank stare you'll get when you tell your daughter that she shouldn't diet because it may contribute to osteoporosis at a point that seems about a million years away to her. But tell her anyway. As parents, we need to be aware of the strong associations between dieting and nutritional intake and do our part to help our teens to understand the connection and avoid unhealthy dieting behaviors. Overweight teens who are engaging in weight control behaviors can incorporate low-fat dairy products into their diets to avoid compromising their calcium intake.

DIETING CAN HAVE HARMFUL PSYCHOLOGICAL CONSEQUENCES

In an early landmark study done in Sweden more than 30 years ago, symptoms reported by teenage dieters included fatigue, increased interest in food, depression, poor school performance, anxiety, loss of zest or interest, and mental sluggishness. Since then, other studies have similarly shown that dieting may affect psychological well-being and contribute to the onset of depression in teens. Dr. Eric Stice and his colleagues studied a group of 1,000 high school girls over a 4-year period and found that initial dietary restraint scores strongly predicted the onset of depression four years later; for each unit increase on a dietary restraint scale, the risk for the onset of major depression increased by 50%.

IT'S NOT <u>BEING</u> OVERWEIGHT THAT GETS US DOWN BUT HOW WE <u>FEEL</u> ABOUT IT

The study of 1,000 high school girls conducted by Dr. Eric Stice and his research team found that although dieting and body dissatisfaction were associated with the later onset of depression, body weight was not, indicating that weight-related attitudes and behaviors were more important predictors of depression than actual body size. We are very quick to talk about how being fat in a thin-oriented society can lead to feelings of depression; *these findings suggest that feeling fat and dieting are more likely to lead to depression in teenage girls.* As parents, we need to be thinking about the impact of dieting on our children's psychological well-being.

DIETING CAN BE DISTRACTING

Dieting can distract teens from having greater thoughts. If they're busy counting calories, they may miss out on thinking about how to build space stations or solve world hunger. Skipping breakfast as part of a diet can impair cognitive abilities and lead to lower academic performance. Although young women have made strides in achieving freedom and equal rights, we still have a way to go. Feminist theories view the promotion of extreme thinness in women as a strategy for weakening the power of women. We cannot afford to have our young women be so hungry or so preoccupied with the number of calories that they are eating that their ability to think is impaired.

Can Anything Be Gained by Dieting (Besides Weight)?

You probably do know a couple of people who have lost weight by dieting, kept the weight off, and feel great about themselves. Perhaps they used the diet as a starting point and then began to adopt patterns of eating and physical activity that could be implemented on a long-term basis. But these people are the exceptions, rather than the rule. And rarely are these people teenagers.

I don't want to discount the benefits that dieting may have for some people. Those who are eating extremely poorly may improve their eating patterns and achieve some weight loss by switching to a healthier plan. A diet plan may be needed for people who need to lose weight quickly for medical reasons, such as surgery, and don't have time for lifestyle changes. Some people feel as though they need a strict regime to get started in making changes in their eating patterns. And there are some people who simply make changes more effectively when they can establish certain rules and regulations; they say this allows them to stop ruminating about the goal of losing weight and just stick to a cut-and-dried routine. This is why diets with lots of restrictions, such as the Atkins diet, are so appealing to some people and lead to short-term weight loss.

But what about long-term weight loss and maintenance? In spite of all of the money being spent and made on diet products, services, and books, there are no data showing that these approaches are effective in long-term change. Doesn't that make you a bit suspicious?

Many of the teens we interviewed were sadder-but-wiser former dieters, and they agreed that nothing much could be gained by dieting. One teenage girl went so far as to call dieting "a figment of people's imagination." Characterizing "going on a diet" as a statement of intent, she said she had used the phrase as something of a mantra to psych herself up, but that "it doesn't work." What does work? "Really focusing on what you're eating, focusing on what you're trying to do to make your body better or healthier." In the wise words of this 16-year-old, when your goals are reasonable, *dieting* exits your vocabulary: "You leave that word behind."

WHAT ABOUT LOW-CARB DIETS?

Low-carbohydrate diets were in vogue when I was a teen, and now they've made a comeback. The cover story of *Time* on May 3, 2004, was "The Low Carb Frenzy," and it stated that $30 billion in sales of low-carb foods were expected in 2004 and that 26 million Americans were on a "hard-core low-carb diet right now." If a low-carb diet means cutting back on foods high in simple sugars such as candy and soda pop, eating fewer fat-laden high-carb foods such as muffins, cakes, and cookies, or avoiding huge portions of pasta (often also piled with butter, cheese, or high-fat sauces), it's fine with me. But if it means severely restricting or eliminating the consumption of foods high in complex carbohydrates, (for instance, baked potatoes or rice), replacing carbohydrates with fat (for example, ordering eggs and bacon for breakfast ... but no fruit, please), or choosing foods that have lower levels of carbohydrates but are equal or higher in calories, then I say stay away! Chapter 8 offers more on the importance of balance and moderation, and Chapter 9 explains why calories and portion sizes are what really count.

The Alternative That Works: Healthy Weight Management

We live in a society that constantly encourages us to overeat and under-exercise. The result is that many people are overweight. So, we do need to adopt behaviors that will help our bodies stay at the weight that is healthiest for each of us. For lack of a more exciting term, I call this alternative to dieting *healthy weight management*. This is what I mean by the term:

> **Healthy weight management:** Eating and physical activity patterns based on general guidelines that are adaptable to different situations and practical on a long-term basis.

Examples of healthy weight management include the following:

- Making dietary changes such as increasing your intake of fruits and vegetables, and whole grains, while decreasing your intake of fats and processed sugars.
- Eating when hungry and stopping when full (paying attention to internal signs of hunger and satiety).
- Eating until comfortably full (not stuffed) and knowing that you can eat again when you get hungry.
- Paying attention to what your body is saying it needs.
- Generally using low-fat products (for example, skim milk) when available, but being willing to use other products when they are not available.
- Eating a bit of everything but having smaller portions.
- Cutting down on soft drinks.
- Using cooking techniques that do not require a lot of added fat (such as broiling instead of frying).
- Generally eating three meals a day with small snacks in between, depending on your hunger level.
- Making fruits or vegetables a part of most meals and snacks.
- Starting each day with breakfast.
- Getting some type of physical activity on most days of the week.

How does healthy weight management differ from dieting? In healthy weight management, eating patterns and physical activity behaviors are based on general guidelines. Deviations from overall guidelines occur, but they don't bring about feelings of guilt and thus don't lead to "going wild." Although you may decide that you're going to eat less processed sugar, it's not a strict rule. This means you can eat a piece of cake without feeling as if you've broken your eating plan, which makes it easier to eat just one piece of cake instead of going on to finish off the whole cake.

If that doesn't clarify the difference, take a look at the comments in the following list.

Things people say when engaging in healthy eating for weight management, not dieting:

"No thanks, I'm full."

"Yes, I'd love dessert. Just a small piece, please."

At the movies: "I'll have a small popcorn with no butter."

At McDonald's: "No, I don't want to supersize it!"

At Subway: "I'll have the six-inch turkey sub on whole wheat bread, with all the vegetables, and some honey mustard sauce."

At any restaurant: "Do you want to split the main course and then share a dessert?"

"I've started walking to school instead of taking the bus. It doesn't take me much longer, and I start off the day feeling better."

"When I got home from school (work) I had an apple and yogurt to tide me over until dinner."

"I try to eat a good breakfast to avoid getting too hungry in the middle of the day."

"I kind of feel like eating, but I think it's due to boredom rather than actual hunger; maybe I'll take a walk first and see how I feel afterward."

"I've discovered a million different ways to eat fruits and vegetables."

"This is delicious. I am really enjoying this meal. But no thanks to seconds."

Clearly, these statements are less self-punishing and more forgiving than those made when dieting. Healthy weight management measures are less likely to have negative consequences for a person's self-esteem. They allow teens to enjoy eating and being physically active and are thus more likely to be helpful for long-term behavioral change.

So how do we know that what I call *healthy weight management* works?

In a study of 3,000 adults who lost a significant amount of weight (an average of 66 pounds) and have kept it off for a number of years (an average of five years), Dr. Rita Wing and her colleagues found that the successful losers report four common behaviors. They eat a low-fat, high-carbohydrate diet, are physically active for about an hour a day, eat meals and snacks (an average of five meals/snacks a day), and do some self-monitoring of their body weight and food intake. Thus they have adopted a pattern of eating and physical activity that's in line with national dietary guidelines and can be used over the long term. They are not engaging in "diets," although they've made significant behavioral changes that have enabled them to lose weight and maintain the weight loss.

In several of our own studies with teenage girls and boys, teens who engaged in healthy weight control behaviors such as increasing fruit and vegetable intake or physical activity were healthier all around than teens eating very little, fasting, or skipping meals. In Project EAT, we found that girls using unhealthy weight control behaviors had lower intakes of fruit, vegetables, grains, calcium, iron, vitamins A, C, and B_6, folate, and zinc than girls using only healthy weight control behaviors. Clearly, it's crucial to distinguish between restrictive dieting practices that can lead to feelings of deprivation and the harmful consequences of that feeling, and principles of healthy weight management that allow for enjoyable eating experiences that may be the bases for lifetime patterns.

WHAT DO TEENS HAVE TO SAY ABOUT ALL THIS?

Dr. Mimi Nichter and her colleagues found that teens make the same distinction between dieting and healthy weight management that we do, although they don't necessarily use this type of language. Among the girls they interviewed, they found two groups of teens who think about weight control—those who "diet" and those who "watch what they eat." The teens said that dieting involves rigid rules, which often set the girls up for personal failure and frustration, but "watching" is a more positive action that allows them to be flexible and negotiate their eating patterns in different situations. Dr. Nichter observed that dieting involves "being controlled" by an imposed structure, whereas watching entails "exerting control." Furthermore, watching involves the broader concept of eating more healthfully as distinct from eating less.

Dr. Nichter found that dieting often does not involve sustained changes, but can, for some girls, last for just a day or two, or even for just a few hours between breakfast and lunch, when they see their friends eating chocolate or french fries. This, of course, may explain why dieting has not been found to be very effective in weight control for most teens. It also explains why it might be associated with weight gain. In our own research we asked teens, "What do you or your friends do when dieting?" One teenage girl echoed the disconnect between intending to diet and actually changing behavior that I mentioned earlier, saying that her friends would say they were dieting and then immediately head off for fast food, justifying their decision by claiming they'd start their diets "tomorrow."

This kind of vacillation between going on and off a diet tells us that teens may lack the skills and support needed to make healthy eating and physical activity part of their everyday lifestyle, which is why they say they're "going on a diet"—it's an expression of the intent to eat healthily without a clue as to how to go about it. This is where you come in.

What You Can Do When Your Teenager Wants to Diet

When your teenage daughter announces at the dinner table that she can't eat anything being served because she's on a diet, what do you do? What do you say when you hear your daughter and her friends talking about how fat they are and about a new diet that they're going to start together? How about when your son says he's decided to give up breakfast to save some calories? How about when he asks for money to buy the latest diet book that promises quick results without pain?

How you will deal with the situation will, of course, depend on your teen and your family, including factors such as your teen's age, your teen's overall eating patterns and weight history, your own dieting and weight issues, your relationship with your teen, and family communication styles. But any of the signs I just described would set off a little alarm in my head: time for some discussion and possibly some other type of action.

I would take a deep breath to avoid overreacting and think about how best to respond. I would check over the 10 guidelines shown on pages 115–117 and think out a game plan. I would be particularly concerned if my daughter (or son) was not overweight, if she had individual characteristics that might increase her risk for an eating disorder (for example, perfectionist tendencies or low self-esteem), if she was immersed in a weight-conscious environment (for instance, involved in a weight-related sport), or if there was a family history of weight-related problems. Regardless of her weight, I would want to explore what was going on that was leading to her desire to diet and what she meant by going on a diet.

However, we also need to remember that teens are in the process of separating from their parents, and a desire to go on a diet may merely be part of this process. If so, you wouldn't want to overreact but might want to work with your teen in figuring out exactly what is motivating her to diet, what her plan is for changing her eating habits, and where you will need to step in if she seems to be taking a wrong turn.

what you can do
SIGNS THAT YOU NEED TO TAKE IMMEDIATE ACTION

A big thing to look for is *change*—change in appearance, emotion, or behavior. Is your daughter suddenly skipping meals? Finding excuses not to participate in family meals? Is she playing with food to make it less obvious that she isn't eating—pushing food around on her plate or cutting it into little pieces? Is your son exercising excessively? Does your teenager persist in expressing dissatisfaction with his or her body shape and size despite having lost weight? Have you noticed any overall mood changes, including social withdrawal, fatigue, nervousness, or irritability? Chapter 15 explains what you can do if your teen has moved toward the problematic end of the spectrum of weight-related disorders and is displaying anorexic or bulimic behaviors.

what you can do
SOMETIMES A SIMPLE RESPONSE IS ALL THAT IS NEEDED

If your child is a preteen or at the young end of adolescence, and you're fairly certain that her expression of interest in dieting is being made without a whole lot of thought or baggage behind it, you might try making a clear statement such as "*In this family we don't diet.*" Sometimes there's nothing like a zero-tolerance statement made with conviction for conveying how important you feel it is to avoid dieting. I still strongly recommend following up with some of the 10 guidelines for action, such as finding out why your teen is interested in dieting, determining whether something else is bothering your teen, and using this as an opportunity to help your child adopt healthier eating and physical activity behaviors.

The following are 10 general guidelines for how to respond when your child says something like "I'm starting a diet tomorrow" or "I feel so fat. I should go on a diet." Please note that not all of this information has to be discussed in one conversation, nor should it. It's kind of like talking about sex; if at all possible, we want to avoid having "the sex talk." Instead, we try to integrate discussions about sexual relations into various conversations over the years. Ideally, discussions about body image, self-acceptance, healthy eating, and dieting should occur at different stages in your child's development. However, if that hasn't been the case so far, don't despair. When the topic of dieting is brought up, explore what's going on in your teen's life and why this interest in dieting has arisen. Leave the rest for another conversation.

1. Clarify why your teenager is interested in dieting. Does something else lie behind the interest in dieting that doesn't have to do with weight? Is your teen feeling insecure? Explore your teen's general feelings of self-worth to see if this concern is really about weight. Sometimes it's easier to blame weight than other, more nebulous problems. One teenage girl we interviewed said she thought kids who talk about dieting feel insecure, that "they don't feel right about something about them." Has your teen been teased because of his or her weight? Explore whether something specific has recently happened, such as being teased or having friends start fat talk. It's important to know if this is the case so you can figure out how best to proceed and help your teen.

2. Compliment and reassure your teen. Reassure your children that you think they look beautiful, remind them about their positive traits, and let them know that you love them. This reassurance should always be given early in any individual conversation about dieting, but it should also be offered later in the conversation and sprinkled throughout. *You can't say these things too often.* If your teen really is overweight and you think weight loss is warranted, the same meaningful compliments and reassurance are important. Advice can come later—for now just let your teen know you're there for him and want to help him out.

3. Address nonweight issues. If the underlying issue isn't really weight, the next step is to make yourself available to talk about the issues that really are troubling your teen. Help your teen understand why it's so easy to focus on weight in a society like ours, where we're taught that being thin will solve most of life's problems. If your teen has been teased about weight, be supportive and let your child know that no one needs to put up with that. If your teen really is interested in dieting, continue with step 4.

4. Clarify what your teen means by going on a diet. Is the idea just to cut down a bit on certain foods? Is the plan more extreme? Is your teen already doing something? If so, what?

5. Discuss the advantages of healthy weight management versus dieting. Talk about the possible dangers of dieting and its ineffectiveness. Discuss the value of paying attention to signs of hunger and not eating in response to other feelings. Discuss the diet–binge cycle. You may want to help your teen reframe her thinking in terms of healthy weight management: "Oh, it sounds as though you're interested in making some changes in your eating patterns and physical activity that can help you achieve the weight that's healthiest for you." Although teens tend to want quick results and aren't interested in the long-term effects, let your teen know that physical activity will help in preventing weight gain over time. It's important to talk about calories and portion sizes, but this needs to be done in a manner that takes into account the sensitivity of teens to these topics; see Chapter 9.

6. Offer to help—but not with dieting. Strongly state that you don't want your daughter to "diet" but you're willing to help her adopt healthier eating and physical activity behaviors. Ask what she'd like from you. How can you help? Make some suggestions, such as making a shopping list or going grocery shopping together, buying some healthy snacks, going for a walk after dinner, signing her up for a hip-hop class, or getting her passes for the local swimming pool. If your teen expresses an interest in weight control, turn the situation into a teachable moment to say some of the things you've been wanting to say about healthy eating, but were afraid to utter for fear of getting the "glazed-over look." Often teens don't care very much about their nutrition, but now you have a perfect opportunity to talk about topics normally considered boring, such as meals, portion size, low-fat dairy foods, whole grains, and vegetables. Chapter 8 contains lots of information on nutrition you can use.

7. Focus on behaviors, not weight. Discuss why it's important to focus on behavioral change and not weight. Reinforce the notion that different people come in different shapes and sizes. We can control what we eat and how much we exercise, and then we need to let our bodies find the weight that is healthiest for us.

8. Acknowledge the difficulties faced in being different. Don't dismiss the difficulties that your teen may be facing if her weight differs from that of her friends or cultural norms. Explore options where your teen may feel accepted and more comfortable, regardless of shape or size. Some teens may find supportive networks outside of school, within religious groups, youth movements, volunteer programs, or summer camps. But do discuss the whole cultural obsession with thinness and the fact that different people have different body shapes. Your teen can be empowered by questioning society's obsession with thinness.

9. Find the balance between over- and underinvolvement. If your teen does decide to diet, avoid getting overinvolved, unless you have concerns about your teen taking things too far. As much as possible, avoid making comments on changes in your teen's weight. If you do want to pay your teen a compliment, focus on positive behaviors and raise concerns about any negative behaviors. For example: "I've noticed that you're eating a salad every night at dinner, which is great. I'm a bit concerned that you're not getting enough calcium and protein, which are so important for muscles and bones. I'm going to add some shredded cheese to the salad. Then you could either have a glass of milk with dinner or some calcium-fortified orange juice. Which would you prefer?" Remember that you can't control your teen's behaviors, but you can control your own behaviors—what you agree to buy, what you're willing to cook, and what you say about your own weight or other people's weight. You can't force your teen to eat more or eat less, to diet more or to diet less, but you can provide an atmosphere that is supportive of the healthier choices.

10. Seek professional help. If you're feeling nervous about guideline no. 9 and trying to decide where the fine line lies, arrange to have your teen meet with a dietitian, a psychologist, or your pediatrician. Your teen may be more likely to listen to someone other than a parent, and the conversation is sure to be less emotional. I would certainly recommend consulting a health care provider if you suspect your teen is taking things a bit too far, or if you have some real concerns about your child's weight and want to take advantage of his or her interest in making changes. However, such a consultation can be helpful even if this is not the situation. A professional who specializes in adolescent health care and who has experience with weight-related issues such as obesity or eating disorders is obviously your best bet, if available. It may be helpful to meet first with the health care provider to see if the relationship will be a good fit and to provide a bit of background information on your teen and your concerns.

what you can do
MINIMIZE USE OF YOUR SCALE

To weigh or not to weigh? This is a question to which you'll get different answers from different people. Many obesity professionals say that prudent use of a scale can help with preventing weight creep over the years. Most eating disorder professionals say, "Get rid of it." My sense is that it depends on age, weight history, and reaction to what you see on the scale. Some people find that having a scale at home just reminds them to go for a walk after lunch if they've put on a little weight. But for others, getting on the scale can lead to a "bad weight day": what they see can affect their mood and feelings of self-worth. For some, it can lead to the use of dangerous weight control behaviors such as the use of laxatives or vomiting. *Getting rid of your scale can make a strong statement to your teens if you're trying to play the focus on weight down in your home and play up behavior.* Think about whether or not you want a scale in your home. If you decide you want to keep it, minimize its use, don't talk about how much you weigh, and never weigh your children . . . leave that for your pediatrician.

what you can do
IT'S NEVER TOO LATE . . .

If you're worried that your teenager's interest in dieting is a product of your own preoccupation with weight, rest assured that you can still make positive changes—for yourself and your teen. Sometimes, in fact, it's easier to make changes in our own behaviors when we see how they might affect our kids. Take gradual steps toward change. Stop talking about dieting. Stop making negative weight-related comments. Share your "mistakes" with your teen (without telling everything) if you think that might be helpful. Buy some foods that are not "diet" or low-fat and eat them in front of your teen. Don't worry that you're acting unnaturally and your teenager will notice. That's exactly what you want, and even small, gradual changes in what you model will have a positive impact on your teen—if not immediately, then over the years to come.

7

The Four Cornerstones
of Healthy Weight and Body Image

What can you do to help your teens avoid excessive weight gain without becoming so preoccupied with getting or staying thin that they develop unhealthy, harmful habits? If you've read the first six chapters of this book, you may already know the answer. All the research you've read about points to four principles that form the cornerstones for a lifetime of healthy eating, positive body image, and life-sustaining activity. These principles serve as your foundation for preventing and resolving weight-related problems in your teenagers. The remaining chapters in this book offer the building blocks that you add as you put the principles into action in daily life.

This chapter gives an overview of the four cornerstones for promoting healthy weight and body image in your teen. Although these cornerstones will provide you with some guidance as to what you can do to help your teen, I don't want to give the impression of oversimplification. We both know how complicated parenting a teenager can be, especially when you have to fight a trend that seems to have the force of a juggernaut and the same magnitude of potential for harm. With this overview, I hope to equip you to make small changes every day that can add up to lasting protection for your teen. In the rest of the book, I'll show you the many ways in which other parents have done this, but you'll have to adapt these approaches to fit the needs and desires of your own family.

THE FOUR CORNERSTONES FOR PROMOTING A HEALTHY WEIGHT AND POSITIVE BODY IMAGE IN YOUR TEEN

1. **Model healthy behaviors for your children.**

   Avoid dieting, or at least unhealthy dieting behaviors.
   Avoid making weight-related comments as much as possible.
   Engage in regular physical activity that you enjoy.
   Model healthy (but not perfect) eating patterns and food choices.

2. **Provide an environment that makes it easy for your children to make healthy choices.**

   Make healthy food choices readily available.
   Establish family meal norms that work for your family.
   Make physical activity the norm in your family and limit TV watching.
   Support your teen's efforts to get involved in physical activity.

3. **Focus less on weight, instead focus on behaviors and overall health.**

   Encourage your teen to adopt healthy behaviors without focusing on weight loss.
   Help your teen develop an identity that goes beyond physical appearance.
   Establish a no tolerance policy for weight teasing in your home.

4. **Provide a supportive environment with lots of talking and even more listening.**

   Be there to listen and provide support when your teen discusses weight concerns.
   When your teen talks about fat, find out what's really going on.
   Keep the lines of communication open—no matter what.
   Provide unconditional love, not based on weight, and let your child know how you feel.

Before you read about these cornerstones, please know that one reason they work so well with teens is that they take into account key processes of adolescent development, namely, the development of a sense of identity and increasing autonomy in relation to one's parents. I probably don't have to tell you that body image and self-esteem tend to be quite intertwined during adolescence. Both contribute to your teenager's developing identity. As you've read in Chapter 4, societal pressures don't exactly work to help teens develop a positive body image. As parents, we play a crucial role in enhancing our children's sense of identity and bolstering their body image and self-esteem. By relying on these four cornerstones you can help your teen achieve a healthy weight without putting the emphasis on weight and inadvertently damaging your child's body image, overall self-esteem, or developing identity.

These cornerstones also allow you to help without interfering with your teen's developing autonomy. When you have a teen at home, the question of who's in control comes up constantly. For example, who should be in control of when, what, and how much teens choose to eat? Teens want to be, and should be, in control of what they eat, but they need parental support in making healthy food choices and developing healthy eating patterns. Your teenagers may develop eating problems if you exert too much control, monitor what they eat too closely, and force them to adopt a preset eating pattern that's not of their own making. But eating problems can also arise if you pull away too soon and too drastically from food preparation or never expect your teens to partake in family meals. As with most issues of adolescence, balance is key, with parents providing the necessary structure and support while teens make the final decisions about how much and what they eat. The pace will vary from family to family, but all families have to gradually transfer responsibility and let go of their teenagers. Following the principles of the four cornerstones can allow you to go a long way toward helping your teenagers develop a healthy weight and body image without issues of control even coming into the picture.

1. Model Healthy Behaviors for Your Children

I won't go into much detail on the foundations for this rule. I'm sure you could have guessed that this would be number one just from reading the first six chapters of this book, in which we saw that teens emulate the behaviors they see around them—particularly among those closest to them. Here's what you're aiming for:

DON'T DIET!

If you don't want your children to diet (which I hope you don't after reading Chapter 6), you shouldn't do it yourself. If you absolutely must diet, do it in a healthy manner and don't talk about it. When offered dessert, instead of saying something like "I can't—I'm dieting," you might want to try something like "I'll have an apple; I haven't had enough fruits and vegetables today" or just "No, thanks." Or when you go to work out, do you ever come home and say something like "I'm working out so much and not losing weight; I don't know if it's worth all the time"? Instead, try something like "I can really tell the difference in my strength and stamina since I've been working out." Up front, you may want to let your family know about your intentions by saying something like "I'm not going on any more 'diets.' Instead I'm going to focus on some long-term changes in my eating and physical activity patterns that can make me feel better about myself."

CAN'T WE TALK ABOUT SOMETHING OTHER THAN WEIGHT?

It's not just our teens who live in a society that associates thinness with beauty, success, and happiness. We do too, and we need to remind ourselves not to get caught up in this frenzy. Hard? You bet! So fake it until you make it. Avoid making any negative weight-related comments about yourself or anyone else in front of your children. Better yet, try not to make any weight-related comments even if none of your children are around. When the topic of weight comes up in conversations with your friends, avoid going there. Avoid the urge to engage in fat talk or to make negative remarks about your body size or shape when your friends make these remarks about their own bodies. Sound hard to do? Here are some examples of the "old" way of addressing friends' comments about weight and an alternative "new" way:

> YOUR FRIEND: I've gained so much weight. I don't know how you stay so thin.
>
> YOUR OLD RESPONSE: Oh my gosh, are you kidding? I've gained so much weight; you just can't tell because I'm wearing black.
>
> YOUR NEW RESPONSE: I think you look great. And you know what? I've decided to stop talking and thinking about weight so much. I'm focusing on eating and exercising for health and for fun!

> YOUR FRIEND: Have you lost weight?
>
> YOUR OLD RESPONSE: No, but I wish I could. I keep trying but it's pretty much hopeless.
>
> YOUR NEW RESPONSE: No.

I recently attended an eating disorders conference where we discussed the question of making weight-related comments to others and whether it was ever appropriate. For example, if a friend loses weight, should you comment on it? Before you do, think about how your friend will feel if she *has* lost weight but then gains it back (as often happens). Or think how you will feel if she loses too much weight because of all the positive feedback that she receives. The other day someone asked me if I had lost weight. She may have meant it as a compliment, but it made me wonder if she thought I *should* lose weight. It reinforced my belief that we need to think twice before commenting on anyone's weight. I'm not saying that it is never appropriate to make a weight-related comment. Sometimes a word of positive reinforcement is absolutely appropriate, such as when a friend has been trying to lose weight after being diagnosed with diabetes. But most of the time it's just better to avoid such remarks. Remember, your children are learning from you.

GET OFF THE COUCH—AND TRY TO HAVE FUN MOVING AROUND A BIT!

So, if you aren't going to diet, what are you going to do instead? Chapter 5 discussed the important role of physical activity in healthy weight management. Get active and make sure your teen sees you doing it. Also try to focus on the benefits of being active other than calorie burning. This is hard to do on a treadmill, but easy to do if you walk around a lake. When you talk to your teens about your own physical activity, put the emphasis on why you like being active and how it makes you feel better. Next time you're heading out for a quick dinner at the local grill, suggest that the family walk there if it's a reasonable distance. If your kids ask why, say, "Because it's beautiful outside and I work indoors all day"—don't say that it's so you'll work off all the calories you're about to consume.

IF YOU WANT YOUR TEEN TO DRINK MILK, DON'T ORDER SODA POP FOR YOURSELF

Take a look at your own eating patterns and food choices. They make a difference to your children. If you eat breakfast, they're more likely to eat breakfast. If you eat fruits and vegetables, they're more likely to do so as well. If you drink milk, they're more likely to drink milk.

Instead of modeling dieting to your teens, model healthy eating behaviors, which are more effective than dieting and have less potential for damage. These include (but are not limited to) portion control (for example, a small container of popcorn at the movies, a six-inch sub at Subway, and no supersizing meal deals), having salad and cooked vegetables at dinner (or at least one of them), and going easy on the added fat and oil (for example, use mustard instead of mayonnaise on sandwiches). You may choose to use low-fat products, although I recommend not going overboard here or making it a religion (if they don't have skim milk for your cappuccino, regular milk won't kill you). I also recommend modeling eating small amounts of dessert (it is possible to have one piece of cake). The key is to do these things without making a big deal of them. Rather than making your choices seem like a sacrifice or self-deprivation, don't comment at all or make a comment that reinforces a behavior you would like your teen to emulate. If your teen asks why you're getting the small popcorn (maybe you used to buy the jumbo popcorn at the movies because it's a better deal), just say you're not that hungry or that you've realized that when you buy the big one you tend to eat past the point of enjoyment. There are more ideas like this in Chapters 8–13.

2. Provide an Environment That Facilitates Healthy Choices

Here's one of the key messages of this book: You can do a lot to prevent all the problems on the spectrum of eating, activity, and weight concerns by creating a healthy and supportive home environment. Easier said than done—I know. We live in crazy times, so even simple things like having dinner together as a family become very complex and in some cases impossible. But we need to know that most teens will reach for potato chips instead of an apple unless it's very easy for them to eat the apple (that is, if it is washed and within a hand's reach). Our society has made it much easier to engage in unhealthy eating and physical activity behaviors than to practice healthy behaviors, so we need to work against the current. Some ideas for providing a supportive structure within your home are provided in the following pages, and the theme is picked up in more detail in the remaining chapters of the book.

HAVE HEALTHY FOOD CHOICES WITHIN ARM'S REACH

One of the best ways to get your children to eat healthy foods is to have them readily available. The teens who participated in our studies talked a lot about eating foods that are easy to find and easy to eat. Take a look in your cupboards and fridge. Do you have washed fruit, cut-up vegetables, dried fruit, yogurt drinks, orange juice, cheese and crackers, and pretzels on hand? Julia, who has no kids of her own but always has a houseful of nieces, nephews, and their friends, keeps a gigantic bowl of ripe peaches, plums, and cherries on her kitchen pass-through counter in summer—and reports that no one ever asks for chips. Cheryl buys bottled water even though she hates the waste of disposable bottles, because if it's cold and in the fridge, her kids will drink it. If they have to wait for the tap water to get cold and to fill up a glass, they're likely to grab a soda pop instead. Don't underestimate the power of putting food in the front of the fridge: Many people, including teenagers, seem to think that if it doesn't leap out at them, it's not in the refrigerator. Keep the fruits, veggies, and yogurt right up front.

I also think it's important to have a variety of foods in your home so that certain items do not become "forbidden" foods. But I suggest greatly limiting the amount of soda pop in your house. Sodas not only contain no valuable nutrients, but they substitute for water, juice, and milk, all of which are much better choices.

MAKE IT EASY FOR YOUR KIDS TO EAT MEALS

Family meals provide a setting for modeling healthy eating patterns, offering healthy foods, monitoring what your children are eating, and interacting with family members. Because family meals are so important and so difficult to make part of daily life, we've done quite a bit of research on family meals in the homes of teens. The ideas that our studies have yielded for increasing the frequency and payoff of family meals can be found in Chapter 11. And since some days are crazy, and we just don't have the time or energy to cook, I've provided some ideas for eating out healthfully as a family in Chapter 12.

It's ideal for all or most family members to eat together, but the least we can do is make sure our teens are eating meals at all. Many don't. Always on the run, they sometimes look at eating as a necessary evil that they fit in only where they can, which often means in the car, on the way somewhere, and too often means fast food. Are your teenagers running out of the house without eating in the morning? Are they out and about in the evening instead of coming home for dinner? What can you do to ensure that they're eating meals? What foods would they like to have at home? What are the family expectations regarding meals and skipping meals? What can be done within your home to make it easier for your teens to eat regular meals? You're the expert on your home and your family, so you know what would work best in your situation. You or your spouse may be willing to get up in the morning and make a hot breakfast for your kids before they leave for school. Or you may prefer to have them write down on a shopping list some quick and easy foods that they can eat on their own, like cereals or frozen waffles. Or you may need to resort to foods they can grab on their way out the door, such as cereal bars or yogurt drinks. The point is that you want to make it as easy as possible for your teens to eat meals, to ensure that they are getting enough to eat, increase their likelihood of having adequate nutrient intake, and minimize the amount of snack food that they might otherwise be consuming.

TURN OFF THE TUBE!

As I said in Chapter 5, children raised in a home in which physical activity is the norm are more likely to incorporate physical activity into their lifestyles. Does your family go out for a walk after dinner, go to a lake or pool on a nice day (and actually swim), get out for a game of tennis, go for a bike ride? When you plan vacations, do you think about doing something active? Where is there room for change? What about sedentary activity? One of the best things you can do is to limit the amount of television watching in your house. Taking into account the nature of teens and their love of rules, you might want to make sure that you don't make this a negative thing ("You can watch only a half-hour of TV on weeknights") but instead just put healthy behaviors in their place (just as in having healthy food available, have alternative activities available).

PROVIDE TRANSPORTATION, FILL OUT FORMS, ETC. . . .
TO SUPPORT YOUR CHILDREN'S EFFORTS TO BE ACTIVE

If you can support your children's efforts to be involved in different physical activities, they're more likely to be active. When we were growing up, this often meant just letting your kids play outside after school. Now things are a bit more complicated, and this may involve driving or arranging car pools, signing up kids for community sports or camps, showing up at their games to provide support, helping them get involved with peer groups that are physically active, helping them find sports that work for them, and providing a lot of encouragement and positive feedback. Your children may not be good enough for the highly competitive leagues, and you may need to look a bit harder for opportunities for physical activity. A friend of mine, as co-chair of the sports committee at her daughter's middle school, took the initiative to establish a program in which the school gym would be open on Sundays for open basketball, a sort of family event. Also, don't hesitate to ask your kids to join you if you're going for a walk, taking a dance class, or lifting weights; this may provide you with some time to talk while being active.

3. Focus Less on Weight; Instead, Focus on Behaviors and Overall Health

So, does all this mean you shouldn't be saying anything? No, not exactly. It means you can do a lot, without saying much of anything, through role modeling and changes in your home environment. It also means that when you do say something, it should focus on behaviors rather than on weight. We've seen how much pressure teens face in regard to weight-related issues. Your teens would have to be walking around with earplugs and paper bags over their heads to be unaware of the intense social pressures to be thin. Therefore, your additional pressure is probably not going to be helpful and any comments you make are likely to be seen as unhelpful and even hurtful.

ENCOURAGE TEENS TO CHANGE THEIR BEHAVIORS; WEIGHT WILL TAKE CARE OF ITSELF

In general, it's much more helpful to focus on behaviors than on weight, because we have more control over behaviors than weight and because eating and exercise behaviors are less sensitive subjects than body shape and size. Since teens already get enough pressure to be thin, the messages you want to get across to your teen are as follows:

- "It's important for your overall physical and psychological well-being to eat healthfully and engage in physical activity."
- "If you do these things, your weight will find the level that's healthiest for you. This may differ for different people, so you may end up at a higher weight than your friends."
- "Beauty comes in different shapes and sizes. The important thing is to take care of yourself at whatever weight you are."
- "I will love you no matter what your size."

It's probably best to wait until your teen brings up her concerns about weight with you. When she does, try to establish whether she's really concerned about her weight or whether something else is bothering her (for example, she was teased at school, she's having relationship problems, and so on). If it

127

really is a weight issue, then comments and questions such as those listed here may be helpful:

DAUGHTER: Mom, I really need to go on a diet.

MOTHER: What's going on?

DAUGHTER: Honestly, nothing has happened. But I've just been thinking that I want to start taking better care of myself. I've gained a lot of weight over the past couple of years, and I want to slow it down a bit.

MOTHER: Well, I think taking care of oneself is important for everyone, regardless of a person's weight. I happen to think that you look beautiful. I also think that beauty comes in different shapes and sizes. There isn't just one body shape that works.

DAUGHTER: Mom!

MOTHER: But I'm certainly willing to try to help you figure out a way to improve your eating patterns and to get a bit more active. What are your thoughts about what might help you make healthier food choices? Are there foods that you'd like me to buy? Should we make a list together?

DAUGHTER: Well, it would probably be good if I could bring some healthy snacks to school so that I don't end up buying things in the vending machines. Also, maybe you could give me and a friend a ride to the gym when you go, and we can lift some weights and walk around the track.

MOTHER: Those are great ideas. I'm going shopping tomorrow, so I'll pick up some healthy snacks, and tomorrow evening we can go to the gym together. Just remember that through healthy eating and regular physical activity, your weight will settle at what's best for you. That might differ from your friends'. The main thing is to focus on doing healthy things; your weight will take care of itself.

DAUGHTER: That's easy for you to say!

MOTHER: I know it's not easy to accept, because we read so much about how we can be any weight we want as long as we work hard enough at it. That's what sells magazines and diet products.

DAUGHTER: Well, let's see what happens.

MOTHER: Sure. Just know that I'm here to help you *do* healthy things, not give things up. I'm proud of you for doing something on your own. And don't forget—your parents will love you no matter what!

HELP YOUR TEEN DEVELOP AN IDENTITY THAT GOES BEYOND PHYSICAL APPEARANCE

It's our job as parents to make sure our teenagers' sense of self does not focus strictly on the physical self. To broaden and enhance your teen's sense of self, encourage him to get involved in activities that make him feel good about what he's doing and not how he looks. Teens involved in sports, book clubs, or volunteer activities will begin to define themselves in terms of these activities and not only in terms of weight and appearance.

Think about how you can counteract the negative influence of the media on body image (see Chapter 4). You know your family best and will decide what, if anything, you want to do in regard to media messages that focus on weight, rather than healthy eating and physical activity, as an outcome. In Chapter 4, I gave lots of ideas from other families and the teens we interviewed and worked with.

Praise your children for characteristics that are not appearance-related, such as personality, reading skills, artistic talents, kindness, or ability to engage others in conversation. They still need to hear compliments on their appearance; some ideas for complimenting them in a manner that may broaden their sense of self are provided below.

| **what you can do** |
| COMPLIMENT YOUR TEENS ON HOW THEY LOOK—JUST NOT *ONLY* ON HOW THEY LOOK |

Body image is still an important component of their developing identity, so remember to provide some compliments about how your teens look. Just don't tie your compliments to negative social pressures that overemphasize a particular body shape as ideal. And, if possible, try to broaden your compliments to bring in aspects other than appearance at the same time. Sound way too complicated? Here are some ideas:

"You look so much like Grandpa; when I look at you it brings back so many great memories."

"I love your laugh; it's just contagious."

"Your hands are so graceful – like a pianist's."

"When you smile, your whole face lights up. It's just beautiful."

"I love the way you hold your head up high – it shows great strength and pride."

"Your movements are so graceful."

"You have a caring, inviting look about you that puts others at ease and attracts them to you."

"You have such a great, unique sense of style. I admire the way you wear what looks great on you instead of what everyone else is wearing."

MAKE YOUR HOME A NO-TEASING ZONE

Our society has made it normative to dislike our bodies, particularly if our bodies do not fit the cultural ideal of beauty, so we need to form a home environment in which different body shapes and sizes are respected. Children absolutely need to feel safe and comfortable in their own homes. Many of the teens we interviewed talked about being teased about their weight at home and how hard it was for them—even if they didn't show it or would treat it as a joke. You may think that the teasing going on in your home is being done in a playful manner and isn't hurting anyone. Or without stopping to really think about it, you may not even realize that weight teasing or weight mistreatment is even happening. Remember that your children are probably either the victims or the observers of weight teasing outside the home; they don't need to hear it at home too. If your children are the perpetrators of weight teasing, it's even more important not to allow it at home since they may assume that joking about someone's weight is okay. Let your family know about what you've been reading; let them know that you've come to realize that teasing someone about weight and appearance can be very hurtful and that from now on in your house it isn't going to be allowed. Talk to your family about the similarities between weightism and racism and help them see the pattern. You may not notice any change immediately, but by role modeling the behaviors you wish to see in your children, discussing why weight teasing isn't okay, and reminding them about the no-teasing home policy when they do make comments, you will be able to provide a more comfortable and supportive environment for your family.

4. Provide a Supportive Environment with Lots of Talking and Even More Listening

Oh, the art of listening . . . of just being there for your children when they need your support and not your advice. As a parent, I am finally starting to get this, even though I still have trouble with the concept since I have such wisdom to share with my teens—if only they would listen! Recently my oldest son, who is at college, told me that he really doesn't want my advice, but if it makes me feel better to give it him, that's fine. I tried to tell him that as a college professor, I am paid by people for my advice . . . but that didn't convince him one bit. Truly, often less is more, and we do need to learn to be good listeners and to just provide the support our teens need as they struggle with weight-related issues and all of the other stuff they have to deal with.

BE THERE TO LISTEN AND PROVIDE SUPPORT WHEN TEENS DISCUSS WEIGHT CONCERNS

In my interviews with overweight teenagers, many kids expressed great appreciation when their parents were supportive listeners after the kids had been mistreated because of their weight. If your child is concerned about his weight or has been a victim of weight mistreatment, it's important first to hear him out, then offer support, and only afterward brainstorm some solutions. One thing that teenagers need to hear is that weight teasing is not okay, nor is it their fault that it happens to them.

WHEN THEY TALK ABOUT FAT, FIND OUT WHAT'S REALLY GOING ON

What does your teen mean when she says she feels fat? Why is she comparing herself only with the girls who have the "perfect" bodies? Is she feeling insecure about something else? Find out if "fat" is really the issue or just the "presenting symptom." Getting a teen to open up is no mean feat, of course; specific ideas for communicating are offered in Chapter 13.

KEEP THE LINES OF COMMUNICATION OPEN— NO MATTER WHAT

One of the biggest gifts you can give your child is open communication. This requires time on your part (often at times when you would rather be sleeping). Frequently, it demands patience and nonjudgmental listening. Even if you and your teen are going through a rough spell with power struggles and arguing, you need to know the importance of keeping the lines of communication open. Your teens need you, even if they don't always show it.

what you can do
RESPECT CLOSED DOORS BUT AIM TO OPEN THEM

Respect your teens' privacy and their closed doors. Try not to take it personally when they confide in their friends instead of you—remind yourself that this is part of the healthy separation process of adolescence. But don't be afraid to knock sometimes to remind them that you are there for them. And keep your own door open for conversation . . . literally and figuratively. Most of the time a gentle knock will be sufficient. At other times you will need to knock loudly to get them to talk with you, such as when you see significant and concerning changes in their eating behaviors (e.g., when a child avoids eating with you, plays with food, etc.); activity patterns (e.g., fidgets, does jumping jacks before showering); social life (e.g., withdraws from friends); or mood (e.g., just seems down). More details on what constitutes a significant and concerning change and how to go about opening up difficult conversations are included in Chapter 13 on communication and Chapter 15 on eating disorders. Communication during the teen years may never have been harder, but it has never been so important.

PROVIDE UNCONDITIONAL LOVE, NOT BASED ON WEIGHT, AND LET THEM KNOW HOW YOU FEEL

When our children are little, we often tell them how smart they are, how cute they are, how beautiful their scribbling is, and so on. We give them lots of hugs and kisses. Much of this praise stops when our children reach adolescence, unless we make a concerted effort to keep it going in a way that is acceptable to our teens. We need to keep giving them compliments, and the majority of those compliments, I hope, will focus on non-appearance-related characteristics or behaviors. We need to help them in their efforts to adopt healthy eating and physical activity behaviors. But we also need to make sure they know that we love them, no matter what their weight.

Taking Steps toward Preventing Excessive Weight Gain without Promoting Unhealthy Weight Preoccupation and Dieting in Our Teens

In the following worksheet, write down two to three changes you would like to make within each of the domains listed. Now put a star (★) next to one change in each domain that you plan to address first. Think about what might be most important and effective for your teen. Also take into account the feasibility of implementing this change. Try to be realistic. If you're curious about what I wrote, take a peek at the filled-in worksheet that follows.

What can you do to role model healthy eating and physical activity behaviors for your children and to take the emphasis off weight issues?

1. _____

2. _____

3. _____

What can you do to make your home environment one in which it is easy for your teens to make healthy food choices and be physically active?

1. _____

2. _____

3. _____

What can you do to help your teens focus less on weight, and more on healthy eating and physical activity behaviors?

1. _____

2. _____

3. _____

How can you enhance communication with your teens about weight-related topics and more general adolescent concerns?

1. _____

2. _____

3. _____

Healthy Weight and Body Image

What can you do to role model healthy eating and physical activity behaviors for your children and to take the emphasis off weight issues?

1. *Avoid making any weight comments about people.*

2. *Go swimming at least once a week and let kids know that I do it because it makes me feel great.*

3. *Pay attention to internal signs of hunger when I eat.* ★

What can you do to make your home environment one in which it is easy for your teens to make healthy food choices and be physically active?

1. *Plan ahead so that we can have family meals with decent food at least four nights a week.* ★

2. *Do not allow televisions in children's rooms, even if we have an extra.*

3. *Go heavy on fruits and vegetables next time I shop and use them before they go rotten.*

What can you do to help your teens focus less on weight and more on healthy eating and physical activity behaviors?

1. *When my children talk about eating and weight, I will bring the conversation back to eating for health (e.g., bones, strength).*

2. *When my son complains about weighing too little, I'll encourage him to focus on the behaviors he's trying to change and remind him his weight will take care of itself.* ★

3. *Next time someone makes a weight joke, remind them that we don't allow weight teasing in our home.*

How can you enhance communication with your teens about weight-related topics and more general adolescent concerns?

1. *When my teens talk to me about issues that are important to me, I'm going to bite my tongue during the first five minutes of the conversation so that I will listen more!*

2. *I am going to make myself more available for talking with my teens and seek them out more.*

3. *I am going to give them compliments more often— try to do at least one a day for something deserving (on some days, I may need to look a bit harder than on others).* ★

"What and how much should teenagers eat?"

8

"I Know How to Diet ... I Just Don't Know How to Eat"

What Teens Need to Know about Nutrition

Shahar's mother wants him to eat more vegetables. She asks him what his favorite vegetables are before going to the grocery store. He smiles and says, "Corn and potatoes." His mother wonders, "Do those really count?"

Maya is hurrying through the house to get to school. Her mother asks if she ate breakfast. Maya says, "I made myself a sandwich and I'll eat it at school." Running out the door, she yells behind her, "I did have a glass of orange juice." Her mother asks herself if she should have gotten up earlier to make some eggs but justifies the fact that she didn't with the thought, "Well, at least she took a sandwich with her."

Tal, a senior in high school, has always gone through favorite-food phases. His current favorite is Funyuns with french onion dip. His mother wonders how much she needs to stretch her imagination to count this combination as grains, dairy foods, and vegetables.

Lior drank way too much Mountain Dew in high school; in fact he may have saved the company from going under. But now that he is a college student living in his own apartment, he seems to be coming around; he usually buys juice instead of pop, rarely buys candy, and cooks meals such as tuna melts, meat loaf, chicken parmesan (when he has the money), and various pasta dishes. He even invited the family to his place for Thanksgiving dinner, which he prepared.

Who are these kids? And who is this mother who seems to be wrestling with questions about the adequacy of her children's eating patterns and making justifications left and right? You guessed it. These are my children—and I'm the mother.

Why am I sharing this bit of information at the risk of making myself look bad? I'm telling you this because I think we need to be honest about how difficult it can be to ensure that our teens develop healthy eating patterns without getting too involved, being overcontrolling, or giving up on our career aspirations, free time, or morning sleep. I'm also telling you this because I want to relieve any stress you may be feeling as you read through some of the key dietary recommendations included in this chapter and see what your teen *should* be eating. I strongly believe we need to aim to meet these guidelines . . . but we also need to accept the fact that perfection is an illusion and that trying to achieve it in our teen's eating patterns is very likely to backfire. I also want to show you that even if your teens wander a bit (as my older son did), if you have laid a healthy base for them, they are likely to come around.

How Much Does Nutrition Really Matter?

If you have teens in the house, you know that *quantity* matters. Yesterday five teenage boys came into the house and attacked the food I had just put away after a huge shopping trip, making me feel as though I had wasted my time organizing it all. Keeping enough food in the house to satisfy teenagers is an ongoing challenge. But so is making sure the food they eat is of good *quality*. Children's growth during these years is second only to the amount they grow during the first year of life. Their nutritional needs are greater during adolescence than at any other time in the life cycle.

During adolescence, your kids achieve the final 15–20% of their adult height, gain 50% of their adult body weight, and accumulate up to 40% of their adult skeletal mass. Inadequate nutrition during this period can delay sexual maturation, slow or stop height growth, and interfere with optimal bone development. In contrast, healthy dietary practices can promote optimal short-term and long-term health. Practicing healthy eating behaviors and participating in regular physical activity can help teenagers achieve healthy body weight and body composition and reduce their risk for obesity. Healthy eating behaviors during adolescence have been identified as essential for:

- Promoting optimal growth and development during this period of rapid change.
- Preventing short-term health problems such as iron deficiency anemia, learning difficulties, undernutrition, obesity, eating disorders, and dental caries.
- Laying the foundation for lifelong health and reducing the risk of chronic diseases such as cardiovascular disease, diabetes, high blood pressure, some forms of cancer, and osteoporosis.

To complicate their nutritional needs, by the time they are teenagers your kids have become unique individuals whose activities and circumstances may call for increased nutrients. If your son or daughter can be included in any of the categories in the table on the next page, your challenge to feed your teen well will be even greater.

What Your Teenagers *Should* Be Eating

The food guide pyramid advocates the following basic principles for healthy eating:

- **Variety:** Eat different foods from among and within the different food groups.
- **Moderation:** Limit intake of foods high in fat and added sugars.
- **Balance and proportionality:** Distribute food from among the food groups in proportion to the shape of the pyramid.

"Pyramid eating" means eating a lot of fruits, vegetables, and grains (especially whole grains); moderate amounts of dairy foods and meats or meat alternatives; and a sprinkling of foods that are high in fat and added sugars. I view pyramid eating as similar to a Chinese meal, with rice on the bottom, covered by a generous serving of stir-fried vegetables, topped with some tofu, chicken, or beef. For a complete pyramid meal, this could be served with a glass of milk and a piece of fruit and a fortune cookie for dessert. In teaching the pyramid concept to children, or in reinforcing its relevance for teens, we

Groups of teens	Key needs and challenges
Teens who participate in sports	• High energy needs. • Practices may interfere with mealtimes. • Pressure to conform bodies to specific shapes and sizes for some sports.
Teens with disabilities or chronic illness such as diabetes	• Conditions such as diabetes demand a fairly rigid eating plan. • Teens may face larger pressures to fit in and be "normal." • Parents and teens struggle with balancing demands of condition with need for teen autonomy from parents and desire to be more like peers.
Pregnant teens	• Particularly high nutrient needs. • May discover pregnancy after first weeks, during which intake of nutrients such as folic acid is crucial. • Low motivation, wanting to eat like friends, and limited finances may make it difficult to meet dietary needs of later pregnancy.
Teens involved in substance use	• Appetite disturbances, erratic eating behaviors, and a stressful situation may make it hard to meet nutrient needs, which may be higher than normal
Teens using weight control behaviors	• Need for higher nutrient density, with more nutrients per caloric intake. • Need appropriate balance of energy intake and expenditure.
Teens with eating disorders	• Many nutritional needs—for example, teens with anorexia nervosa have bones in need of calcium to avoid early osteoporosis. • Diet plan in which "forbidden foods" are gradually introduced can be challenging.
Overweight teens	• Feel so much pressure to lose weight that they may not be concerned about nutritional adequacy of intake. • Parents and health care providers may falsely assume that overweight teen is "well-nourished."

sometimes make pyramid parfaits that include all pyramid pieces except vegetables; granola or oats on the bottom of a cup, topped with fruit, yogurt, a few nuts or seeds, and a sprinkling of chocolate chips.

You may be wondering about the wisdom of using the food guide pyramid as your nutritional guide in light of recent updates to the pyramid. If it keeps changing, doesn't that mean that it isn't scientifically sound? Actually, the new 2005 food guide pyramid below continues to promote similar principles to the earlier food guide pyramid, with which your teen may be more familiar. One of the major improvements in the new food guide pyramid is that it allows for more personalization, as reflected in its name, "My Pyramid." This increased personalization is probably a result of:

1. More attention being paid to obesity prevention and the need for a tool that makes different caloric recommendations based on a person's age, gender, and level of physical activity.
2. Enhanced technology that allows people to use an interactive website (*www.mypyramid.gov*) that provides detailed information on dietary needs, serving sizes, different food options, and caloric information.

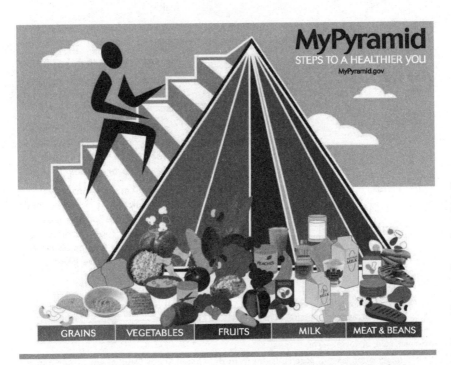

Food guide pyramid: A guide to daily food choices.

Pyramid Eating for Teens

Examples for 16-year-old girls and boys who engage in 30–60 minutes of physical activity a day*

	Girl	Boy	Comments
Calories**	2,000	2,800	
Grains	6-ounce equivalents	10-ounce equivalents	Make half of your grains whole.
			1-ounce equivalent is about 1 slice bread, 1 cup dry cereal, or ½ cup rice or pasta.
Vegetables	2½ cups	3½ cups	Have vegetables from different subgroups: dark green, orange, starch, dry beans and peas, other.
			1-cup equivalent is 1 cup of raw or cooked vegetables or 2 cups of raw, leafy vegetables.
Fruits	2 cups	2½ cups	Eat a variety of fruits and make most choices fruit, not juice.
			1-cup equivalent is 1 cup of fruit or fruit juice or 1/2 cup of dried fruit.
Milk	3 cups	3 cups	Choose fat-free or low-fat most often.
			1½ ounces cheese = 1 cup milk.
Meat and beans	5½-ounce equivalents	7-ounce equivalents	Choose lean products. Vary choices with more fish, beans, peas, nuts, and seeds.
			1-ounce equivalent is 1 ounce meat, poultry, or fish, 1 tablespoon peanut butter, ½ ounce nuts, ¼ cup dry beans or peas.
Other/Extras	Allowance for oils: 6 teaspoons/day.	Allowance for oils: 8 teaspoons/day.	Discretionary calories may include higher-fat or sweetened versions of the food groups above; other foods; or just more from the food groups above (for example, have more grains).
	Limit extras (solid fats and sugars) to 265 calories/day.	Limit extras (solid fats and sugars) to 425 calories/day.	

*Go to the website below for more specific information and to personalize information based on gender, age, and physical activity level.

**Actual calorie amounts may differ in accordance with individual needs and desire to maintain, gain, or lose weight.

Source: Information on this page is drawn from the United States Department of Agriculture's website on the 2005 Food Guide Pyramid: *www.mypyramid.gov*.

The graphics, and some of the recommendations, of the 2005 food guide pyramid are also a bit different from the earlier one, reflecting an increased concern with obesity, gains in scientific knowledge, and common misinterpretations of the previous version of the pyramid. The individual climbing a staircase up the side of the pyramid shows how important it is to be physically active and also shows how we can make changes little by little (one step at a time) to be healthier. In the new graphic, food groups are shown vertically instead of horizontally. The thickness of the wedges portrays graphically which food groups should be consumed in greater amounts. The wedges get thinner at the top of the pyramid, suggesting that not all foods are created equal within food groups. Thus, within the grains food group, a whole wheat slice of bread would be down at the base of the pyramid where the food group is wider, showing that we should be eating more whole grains. A muffin, because of its higher fat and sugar content, would be up at the top of the pyramid where the food group strip is much narrower, showing that we should be eating fewer muffins.

On the facing page I've provided an example of how eating according to the food guide pyramid might work for a moderately active 16-year-old girl and boy. A teenage girl who engages in physical activity for 30–60 minutes a day needs to eat about 2,000 calories a day to maintain her weight. While 2,000 calories provides a point of reference, it is extremely important to note that this number may vary from one girl to the next in accordance with factors such as level of physical activity, movement throughout the day, stage of physical development, body weight, and body composition. The recommendations are for 6 servings of grains, 2½ cups of a variety of different types of vegetables, 2 cups of fruit, 3 cups of milk or equivalent servings of dairy foods, and 5½ ounces of meat and beans. You will find it very helpful to go to the website to get more information on what constitutes a 1-cup or 1-ounce equivalent. For example, one large orange equals a cup of fruit. Of interest is the last row in the table entitled "other/extra." The 2005 food guide pyramid discusses discretionary calories. For these discretionary calories, teens can choose foods such as cookies, potato chips, or ice cream. Or teens can choose to have more of the foods described within the food groups such as more grains. A colleague of mine, Dr. Marcia Herrin, who does a lot of nutritional counseling with overweight teens, has found this concept of discretionary calories to be very useful for teens since it leaves the decision making up to them.

This seems like a lot of food, doesn't it? The point is that if teens limit the amounts of foods high in fats or sugars, they can eat a lot of food. That doesn't mean not eating *any* food high in fat or sugar; it means not making these foods the mainstay of a teenager's diet. Still, 2½ cups of vegetables sounds like a lot more vegetables than most teens are eating. Given the types of foods being served in their environments (home, school, fast-food restaurants) and their food preferences, it's no simple matter to increase the amounts of fresh produce they eat and reduce the amount of fat and sugar. I'll give you some straightforward ways to make the shift a little later.

The food guide pyramid makes plain good sense in promoting variety, moderation, and balance in food choices. Although food fads come and go, we always come back to some type of food-group categorization system (whether in the shape of a rainbow, circle, square, hand, or pyramid) that promotes these principles. Research shows the importance of a diet rich in fruits, vegetables, complex carbohydrates, fiber, and dairy foods and low in saturated fats and refined sugars, for the prevention of a range of conditions including obesity, cancers, cardiovascular disease, osteoporosis, and dental caries. The food guide pyramid has been designed to promote such a diet. As new research becomes available, we will probably see additional modifications in dietary recommendations. But the basics of healthy eating are likely to stay the same. We need to stay away from fads that promote the elimination of entire food groups* (e.g., dairy foods, grains), overemphasize the importance of one nutrient over others and encourage consumption far beyond recommended amounts (usually through supplements), or make promises that sound "too good to be true." Instead, we need to focus our efforts on helping our youth make healthful food choices that are sensible and based on sound science.

What Your Teenagers—and You—Are Up Against

Research shows that between half and three-quarters of teenagers consume less than the recommended amounts of a variety of foods and nutrients. In Project EAT we found that:

- 70% of teenage girls and 57% of teenage boys consumed less than the recommended amount of calcium (1,300 mg of calcium or the equivalent of three to four servings of dairy foods a day).
- 68% of girls and 71% of boys ate less than five servings of fruits and vegetables a day.

---

*Of course, there are individuals with special medical conditions such as lactose or gluten sensitivity or intolerance, who do need to reduce or eliminate certain foods from their diets and find suitable substitutes.

- 48% of the girls and 55% of the boys were getting more than the recommended maximum 30% of their calories from fat.
- 55% of the girls and 64% of the boys were getting more than the recommended maximum of 10% of their calories from saturated fats.

Reversing these trends isn't easy. The fact is that teens just aren't much concerned about long-term outcomes of current behavior, a fact confirmed by my colleagues Drs. Mary Story and Michael Resnick. In their study, teenagers acknowledged the importance of healthy eating practices but said they'd worry more about it later in life—they had other priorities right now. Many teens involved in Project EAT said they would probably eat healthier—if only they had time. This is where we parents usually come in, but making sure teenagers do the right thing isn't as easy as it is with younger kids. We have to be sensitive to their quest for independence.

How Much Should You Try to Control What Your Kids Eat?

Should you allow junk food in your house? Should you say anything when your daughter serves herself another heaping bowl of pasta? What should you do when your son takes a second or third helping of birthday cake? Some of the teens whom our research team interviewed said their families served very healthy meals and kept only healthy foods on hand for snacks. As a result, they admitted, they really enjoyed seeking out something they defined as "incredibly bad for me" when away from home. Why don't they stick to the same pyramid guidelines away from home as they do when they are with Mom and Dad? Maybe it's a matter of too much control.

| **what you can do** AVOID MAKING ANYTHING A "FORBIDDEN" FOOD | Surround your family with healthy food choices, but have some of the "other stuff" available to avoid making them "forbidden foods." Trying too |

hard to control what your children eat can backfire, and they may end up "cheating" or "sneaking" when you're not around.

Dr. Leann Birch and her colleagues followed 140 girls ages 5–9 to see whether early parent feeding practices—how much the mothers said they felt they needed to control their daughters' eating patterns—influenced the girls' eating patterns five years later. To see which girls ate when not hungry, they gave the girls a generous lunch and then offered snack foods. Only the girls who ate a full lunch and said they weren't hungry after lunch were included in the analysis. *Girls whose mothers tried to restrict their intake actually ended up eating more snack food in the absence of hunger when their mothers were not around.* Furthermore, girls who were overweight, and whose mothers tried to restrict their intake, ate the most snack foods. These findings suggest that parental food restrictions can indeed backfire!

Improving Your Teens' Nutritional Intake— Without Becoming a Short-Order Cook

Because of all the research you've been reading about, I've made some changes in my home to promote better nutrition for my kids (with benefits to my husband and me as well). These steps are described below and in more detail in the chapters that follow. Although they haven't produced perfection (or a desire for it) in our family, these changes have made a difference in my children's eating patterns as well as in family and interactions and relationships. Shahar has expanded his vegetable repertoire to include carrots and cauliflower. Tal is snacking more on turkey sandwiches and smoothies and less on Funyons. My kids know they need to join us at the table for dinner if they're home and to keep any "absolutely essential" phone calls very brief during dinner. They all make it a priority to be home for dinner on Friday night (unless something very special, like a big Timberwolves game, is going on) because the food is good and it's just nice to hang out together. And as I said at the beginning of the chapter, my college-age son, Lior, invited us all to his place for Thanksgiving dinner and made quite a spread, including turkey with gravy, cranberry sauce, sweetened cooked carrots, and fancy potatoes with lots of garlic and olive oil. We didn't have to do anything (except pay for the turkey).

I. MAKE HEALTHY FOOD CHOICES THE EASY CHOICE

I couldn't have said it any better than one teenage boy in one of our focus groups: "I have two choices [about dinner at home], take it or leave it. So I take it."

If you want to implement only one guideline, make it this one: *Make healthy foods that are easy to prepare readily accessible.* Or, more bluntly: *Just buy it and put it out.* This doesn't involve overstepping your role as a parent of teens or any nagging, and it doesn't mean offering such foods to the exclusion of less healthy treats. But if you make it easy for them to eat the healthy stuff, your teens will eat it—and they may actually appreciate your efforts. In our research we've found that food availability is the strongest influence on teen eating patterns. In focus group discussions, teens said having healthy foods easily available made them more likely to eat them, particularly foods that don't involve much preparation and cleanup. Foods that can be eaten on the run are also attractive— a lesson the fast-food joints have learned well. Many of the teens said they ate food because it was there in front of them. They'll drink orange juice in the morning if it's already made, but not if they have to mix it. They'll eat healthy food when they don't have to search the cupboard for it. Here are some ideas:

- Have foods such as yogurts, bottled orange juice, bananas, apples, and breakfast bars that teens can eat on those rushed mornings when breakfast just isn't going to happen.
- Most teens come home from school very hungry and have an after-school snack. Many parents aren't around at that time. Have healthy snack foods available such as fruit, carrot sticks, crackers and cheese, pretzels, popcorn, breakfast cereal with milk, and food for making sandwiches such as bagels and cream cheese, rolls and turkey, and tortillas and cheese.
- Cut up the watermelon, put washed fruit in the front of the fridge or on the counter, and put carrot sticks and sliced peppers on the table for nibbling before dinner when everyone is starving.
- Although it takes more than a minute, if you have bananas and frozen berries on hand, your kids might be motivated to make themselves a smoothie.
- Have some cans of chickpeas or dried peas around for snacking. In my fridge, we always have hummus for spreading on bread or using as a dip for carrots.
- Have some healthy frozen entrées available for your teen to snack on after school. Bagel bites and veggie burgers usually go over well with hungry teens.
- Buy extra orange juice and milk when you go shopping so that you don't run out. Put these drinks in a place where teens see them first thing when they open the fridge.

THEY EAT WHAT'S IN FRONT OF THEM

Project EAT showed that you can have a huge influence on the types of foods your teens eat just by buying them and putting them where they'll practically trip over them. Said one boy, "My parents have healthy food on the table, so I just eat what they have."

In our research, we found that having fruits and vegetables at home and serving them at meals was more likely to be associated with teens' fruit and vegetable intake than any other factors, including taste preferences. In homes in which fruit was always available, teens consumed an average of 0.72 more servings of fruit a day than teens in homes in which fruit was rarely available. Similarly, when milk was served at dinner on a regular basis, teens ate an average of 0.79 more servings of dairy food a day than teens in homes in which milk was rarely served at dinner. Conversely, when soda pop was usually available at home, teens consumed an average of 0.87 fewer servings of dairy food a day.

2. GET YOUR KIDS INVOLVED WITHOUT GIVING UP THE SHIP

As teenagers become more autonomous, they need to be involved in the planning, purchasing, and preparation of food, but you need to stay involved too. Here are some ideas:

- Sit down with your teens and ask what kinds of food they would like for snacks and for meals. This makes them feel appreciated, helps you in planning, and somewhat obligates them to eat what you make.
- Keep a running shopping list on the fridge that the kids can add to. You can put limits on what they can add, and certainly on what you will actually buy, but try to go along with reasonable requests. (This way, when they whine, "There's nothing to eat in this house," you can just tell them to write what they want on the list.)
- Consider having a petty cash fund that teens can use to go to the supermarket and buy certain foods on their own (with some restrictions).
- Decide on family expectations regarding your teens' presence at family meals. It's usually okay to insist that they be at the table if you've prepared a meal, but they should know up front that this is an expectation.

- Children also need to contribute to setting up for meals and cleaning up afterward—but it's nice if they can also do the "fun stuff" associated with meal preparation. Maybe Tuesday can be kids' cooking night. Or on a more sporadic basis, ask your kids to help out with some of their "specialties"; in our house that means things like jazzing up the jarred spaghetti sauce, making chocolate balls, blending smoothies, making crepes, grilling when it's nice outside, preparing quesadillas, and making matzo pizza on Passover. Or get them involved in cooking up a dish that you recently ate at a restaurant; on one vacation we had fondue, and all the kids got involved with deciding how we should make it at home.

3. PLAN AHEAD AS MUCH AS POSSIBLE

If you have time to shop and cook every day and enjoy doing this, you can skip this guideline. If not, these tips can be very helpful.

- Get everyone's input and plan at least a few dinners ahead, then go shopping once a week.
- Plan two weekly meals that require some preparation, and make larger amounts for eating on the next day or freezing.
- For other meals, either eat leftovers or make them incredibly easy ones (such as grilled cheese and canned tomato soup, turkey sandwiches with carrot sticks, spaghetti with a bagged Caesar salad, or fried eggs and toast with a salad of chopped cucumbers and tomatoes). Serve milk or orange juice as a drink.
- Make a pot of soup once a week to enhance other meals or be eaten on its own with some bread and cheese or with a salad.
- Think about how to incorporate more legumes and whole grain products into your family's repertoire: make pea soup, add chickpeas to your salad, buy whole wheat buns, and try brown rice.
- Use convenience foods, but stick to those with little added fat or sugar. Go ahead and buy that rotisserie chicken in the supermarket. Frozen vegetables cooked with a bit of soup powder work great. Make use of the salad bar at the supermarket.
- Plan to pick up foods on the way home from work or include eating out in your schedule when things look too crazy for anything else or you just feel like it (see Chapter 12).

I know I've said it before: Modeling healthy eating patterns can really make a difference:

- The dietary guidelines in this chapter apply to you too. How can you make small changes in your own eating in the direction of following the food pyramid?
- Replace weight control measures with measures taken to meet the dietary guidelines. The two complement each other anyway.
- Make changes gradual so as not to get discouraged. If you hardly ever eat whole grains, start by eating a whole grain cereal, whole grain toast, or a whole grain bagel for breakfast.
- Consider eating with your children at breakfast instead of grabbing something to eat at work. Drink a glass of milk instead of a can of soda in front of them. What they see you do has the strongest impact.
- Eat a piece of cake or a small chocolate bar without making negative comments afterward (such as, "I feel so bloated.") or going overboard (for example, eating the whole cake). Instead, comment on how good it is; enjoyment of foods at the top of the pyramid, in moderation, is important and fun.

5. HAVE A VARIETY OF FOODS AT HOME

Designating certain foods as "forbidden" by banishing them from your home sends all the wrong messages to impressionable children and teens. It's overall eating patterns that matter, not a single item consumed on one occasion. Labeling certain foods "bad" and considering themselves "good" if they abstain entirely is a common characteristic of those with anorexia and bulimia nervosa. And as explained in Chapter 6, forbidding eating in general or individual foods in particular sometimes leads to binge eating in teenagers. I've heard stories of families not buying any "extras," or keeping the "good stuff" hidden or even locked up, in the interest of helping their overweight children with weight loss. This is an example of being overcontrolling. It's not only likely to be ineffective, but can have a devastating effect on your child. Please don't do this! Instead try the following:

- If you have overeaters at home, avoid buying the large sizes of snacks, such as the big bags of potato chips. Instead, buy the smaller-portioned bags made for school lunches. This makes it a bit easier to judge portion sizes.
- Don't hide the less healthy food items, but don't make them as accessible as the healthier foods. For example, put some fruit on the counter, but put the chips in a cabinet.
- Take a look at your shopping cart when you get to the cashier in the supermarket. Does your cart reflect the food guide pyramid, with lots of whole grains, fruits, and vegetables; a moderate amount of dairy foods and foods high in protein and iron such as meat, fish, chicken, beans, nuts, or eggs; and a few fun foods such as those higher in fats and sugars?

6. SHOOT FOR GRADUAL CHANGES

Please, please don't despair even if your teens never eat whole grains and dislike most vegetables. Don't shut this book because your family's eating patterns are so far from what you would like them to be that you can't even see the light. Shoot for gradual changes in your home food environment and in your teens' eating behaviors.

- Choose one or two of the preceding guidelines to try out.
- Gradually introduce foods that aren't very well liked, and be discreet about it. One teen actually advised his parents to "include vegetables in every meal—just kind of hide them."
- Stop buying soda pop. Instead drink tap water with ice, bottled water, orange juice, or milk. Easy to do and makes a huge difference. Although juice has a similar calorie content to that of soda pop, and you shouldn't go overboard with it, you get a lot more nutrients per calorie. (In fact, in soda pop you basically don't get any nutrients with the calories.) We'll talk more about calories and how to talk, and not talk, about them in the next chapter.
- Buy the fruit at the supermarket that is already washed and sliced, if fruit in your house that isn't washed and cut up gets thrown away.
- Make a big pot of soup once a month—or once a year. If nothing else, it makes your house smell like real cooking is going on.
- Count potatoes and corn as vegetables (but you'd be stretching things to count the onions in french onion dip).

MAKE HEALTHIER FOOD CHOICES: ONE STEP AT A TIME ...

Instead of ...	Try ...
Cocoa Puffs or Fruity Pebbles	Total or Raisin Bran
A doughnut for breakfast	A whole wheat bagel
Three tablespoons of cream cheese on a bagel	One tablespoon
A cheese and ham omelet	Adding vegetables to the omelet
A side dish of bacon or pancakes	Whole wheat toast or fruit
Snacking on a cookie	Snacking on fruit yogurt
Potato chips	Pretzels or popcorn
A "fruit" roll-up	The real thing—a piece of fruit
A glass of apple juice	An apple (more fiber and more filling)
French fries	Baked potato
Fried chicken	Broiled chicken
Drinking soda pop at dinner	Having a glass of milk
Mocha, frappo, or caramel coffee	Skinny (or regular) cappuccino
Eating a large bag of Funyons	Eating a small bag
Using all the dressing that comes with a salad	Using half as much
Adding meat to the lasagna	Adding spinach
Serving just burgers	Putting out sliced vegetables too
Just buying a cantaloupe	Cutting it into slices
Serving cake for dessert	Putting out the sliced cantaloupe

Adolescent Nutrition:
Making It a Win–Win Situation

Answer the following questions to cement your commitment to make gradual change toward better nutrition for your teen—and your family.

1. What is one dietary change that you would like to see your teen implement? (for example, increase intake of vegetables, other than french fries, to at least one serving a day)

   _____

   _____

   _____

   _____

2. What will you do to increase the chance of this happening without saying a word? (for example, buy V8 juice, make tomato soup for dinner, put out sliced peppers at dinner for nibbling, buy small bags of carrots for eating on the run, model eating vegetables at dinner)

   _____

   _____

   _____

   _____

3. What will you say to your teen to help this happen? (for example, "I'm planning some meals for this week and going grocery shopping tomorrow. What kinds of vegetables would you like me to buy for snacking or for dinner?" or "Please write on our shopping list at least one vegetable that you want me to buy," or "I'm concerned that you're not eating enough vegetables; can you give me some ideas about vegetables that I can buy?")

   _____

   _____

   _____

   _____

What Teens Need to Know about Nutrition

9

Portion Control
and Calorie Counting
Teaching Teens to Pay Attention without Obsessing

Gary orders a supersized burger, large fries, and a milkshake for lunch. His father, who has just been through Weight Watchers, is silently counting up the calories, debating whether he should say something.

Liora takes a look at the restaurant menu, then pulls out a small calorie counter book from her backpack to check a couple of items before making her choice. Her mother is tempted to take a peek herself but doesn't want to reinforce her daughter's calorie-counting behavior, which she thinks is getting to be excessive.

When Sophie's mother cooks, she tries to make enough for at least one day of leftovers. At dinner, Sophie reaches across the table and puts a heaping second serving of spaghetti and meatballs on her plate. Her mother wonders what she can do to help her daughter cut down on portion sizes.

Stuart has told his mother he's interested in losing weight, and she has talked with him about the advantages of thinking in terms of healthy weight management instead of dieting. When they go to a movie together, he orders a large popcorn but tells the counterman to go easy on the butter. Should his mother tell him that he may have just surpassed the pyramid's recommendation for a whole day's worth of grains with that order of popcorn?

Here's where we get to the nitty-gritty. We've been looking at ways to encourage overall healthy eating habits from a variety of broad angles. But now you're sitting at the table with your teenager, and there's no getting around it: You need to address the issue of *how much your son or daughter should eat.*

It's a sensitive topic. A suggestion to take a pass on that second helping of pasta or to order a smaller container of popcorn is likely to be taken as criticism by your child. Your good intentions to help a teen who is struggling with his weight may leave him feeling ashamed of his appetite. And shaming kids, any authority will tell you, is the worst possible way to elicit change. On the other hand, reassurances that your teen doesn't need to count calories at every meal can easily invite adolescent scorn: "But I thought you said we should watch what we eat, Mom. . . . " So what *do* you do?

If you've already come up with the sensible thought that you can solve the dilemma of how much is just enough by serving moderate portion sizes at home, you're off to a good start—as long as you set that example without any verbal fanfare. But it's not likely to be the whole answer. If this involves a change for your family, it won't go unchallenged. And your teens are going to need to know what to do about the huge portions they're likely to be served outside your home, so they'll need to acquire some skills in portion control that they can and will use on their own. But most challenging of all, you're still going to have to find a way to instill awareness of the appropriate amount of food to eat without fueling obsessions over how much to eat.

Calories Count . . . But Don't Count Them

In developing nutrition programs for teenagers, my colleagues and I have had many discussions on this topic. Should we focus only on paying attention to internal signs of satiation in deciding how much to eat, or do teens need information on portion sizes? Dare we even mention the "C" word? We decided to ask teens for their advice in regard to talking about calories. Their responses highlighted two points:

1. *Teens admit they need information.* They want to make informed decisions, and many don't understand the fundamental fact that calories, in and of themselves, are not "bad" but, rather, are needed to live.

2. *They want it delivered respectfully and sensitively.* The teens told us they don't want information to be given in a way that would make them feel bad about themselves—that is, guilty about eating "too many" calories. They wanted us to know that we need to be cautious about saying things that might lead teens to "count calories" and become obsessed with them. They stressed that some teens are more susceptible than others.

You may find it helpful to first get a sense of how much your teen knows about calories and portion sizes.

WHAT IS YOUR TEEN'S CALORIE IQ?

Ask your teen the following questions.

Does your teen have a clue?

1. What has more calories? (a) water or (b) nondiet soda pop
2. What has more calories? (a) whole milk or (b) skim milk
3. What has more calories? (a) a small order of fries or (b) a large order of fries

Knowing the right answers is proof that your teen stayed awake for at least one health class at school. If your teen answers incorrectly, you definitely need to be talking more about nutrition at home. Check out one of the teen nutrition books in the Resources section at the end of this book. [Correct answers; 1 (b), 2 (a), 3 (b)]

Does your teen know enough?

1. What has more calories? (a) a gram of fat or (b) a gram of carbohydrate
2. Which pasta sauce has more calories? (a) marinara sauce or (b) cream sauce
3. About how many calories are in a 20-ounce bottle of cola? (a) 20, (b) 200, or (c) 2,000

(cont.)

The problem is that when we start counting calories, we can become obsessed with them. We can make food choices based on caloric intake without giving thought to other areas of importance such as satiety-producing effects or nutrient density. I remember thinking, as a teen, "Oh, I'll have a chocolate bar instead of a sandwich since it has fewer calories." The problem was that in an hour I would be hungry again. Plus, the sandwich could have supplied a lot more nutrients per calorie than a chocolate bar.

Lucky for us, there are alternatives that we can stress to distract teens from calorie counting.

NUTRIENT DENSITY AND ENERGY BALANCE

A 20-ounce soda pop from a vending machine has about 200 calories with virtually no nutrients. A snack that includes a glass of low-fat milk with an apple also has about 200 calories—but it has 9 grams of protein, 300 grams of calcium, 4 grams of fiber, and a range of other vitamins and minerals. What makes more sense? Talk to your teens about choosing foods for nutrient density, the amounts of nutrients per calorie.

Also talk about calories in terms of their energy intake–expenditure balance. Try explaining it this way to your teenager: "Our bodies need energy, even just for things like breathing. Calories are simply a measure of the energy in the food we eat. You're still growing, so your body needs more energy, but once you stop growing, you'll need less. When you are more active, such as during the soccer season, you need more energy, but during the winter when you're not doing a sport, you need less. It's a matter of balance."

Portion Sizes: Should We Really Be Eating Eight Servings of Grains in One Plate of Pasta?

"I think you've had enough to eat."

"One serving of mashed potatoes is enough; now eat your salad."

"No, you can't have another slice of pizza. Too much pizza isn't good for you."

"You're not hungry? But I made your favorite foods. You need to eat."

"The serving sizes are so big at this restaurant. I suggest we share."

4. About how many calories do most teens need each day? (a) 200–300, (b) 2,000–3,000, or (c) 20,000–30,000
5. Which food has more nutrients per calorie (or a higher nutrient density)? (a) orange juice or (b) Kool-Aid
6. Does a gram of protein have the same number of calories as a gram of carbohydrate? (a) yes, it has the same, (b) no, it has more, (c) no, it has fewer

If your teen knows most of these answers, leave the topic alone. Your teen probably has a good idea of calories and you don't want to push things too much. [correct answers: 1 (a), 2 (b), 3 (b), 4 (b), 5 (a), 6 (a)]

Does your teen know too much?

If you ask your teen how many calories are in 10 peanut M&M's and she answers 103, she knows too much. It is very likely that she has gone overboard with calorie counting. If you hear her say things like "The Krispy Kreme Chocolate Iced Glazed doughnut has 250 calories in it, but the Caramel Kreme Crunch doughnut is even worse and has 350 calories," you should be concerned. If she knows the *exact* number of calories in pretty much *any* food—"An order of six KFC honey barbecued pieces has 607 calories"—check out the list below as well as Chapter 15 to see if your teen is displaying other signs of concern.

Once you know how well informed your teenager is, you need to figure out how susceptible he or she is to putting too much emphasis on weight control measures like calorie counting.

what you can do	Is your teen:
PLAY DOWN THE NUMBERS IF YOUR TEEN IS LIKELY TO TAKE CALORIE COUNTING TOO FAR	➔Already self-conscious and unhappy with his weight and appearance?

➔A picky eater? In this case, he doesn't need another excuse not to eat certain foods.

➔Not overweight? Counting calories when you have no apparent reason to lose weight at all is a warning sign for disordered eating.

➔Exposed to lots of weight talk?

Or have you seen the following behaviors in your teen:

→Makes comments like "I can't eat that; it has too many calories."

→Keeps a list of how many calories she has eaten that day.

→Carries around a purse-size book listing the calories of various foods.

→Reads food labels pretty intensely for the calorie content of foods.

→Measures out foods, such as breakfast cereals, to have, for example, exactly ¾ cup.

→Weighs food to figure out the number of calories being consumed.

If any of the above apply to your teen, *stop talking about calories.* Instead, focus on nutrient density (the amounts of nutrients per calorie), overall nutrition (eating according to the food guide pyramid), eating when hungry and stopping when full, or just eating because it tastes good and is fun.

CALORIES: THE SHORT COURSE

Much of what teenagers hear about calories leads many to believe that *calorie* is a dirty word. Kids need to know what the word means. Start by stressing the idea that unless they consume sufficient calories, they won't have the energy to do the things they want to do. Emphasize balance: *too* many calories will cause weight gain and other health problems, and too few will cause weight and energy loss, which have their own concomitant health problems. All teens need *some* information about the number of calories in various foods so that they don't inadvertently eat way too much or way too little. But no teenager should be encouraged to count the calories in everything eaten or to make a chart or another kind of record. That only makes them worry about calories all the time. Remember this motto: *Calories count . . . but don't count them.*

• Calories are a measure of energy. Without energy, we cannot walk or talk. Thus, calories are not "bad"; they are a measure of something we need to live.

• Weight control depends on a balance of energy intake and energy expenditure. If our caloric intake (what we eat or drink) equals our caloric expenditure (what we use for physical activity, growth, and regular bodily functions), our weight remains the same. If our caloric intake exceeds our caloric expenditure, we gain weight. If our caloric intake is less than our caloric expenditure, we lose weight.

• A pound of body fat has about 3,500 calories of potent[ial]

• If you take in 500 calories less than you expend each day, y[ou] about 5 pounds of body weight in 35 days, or about 50 pounds in [] like many adults, you've gained an extra pound or so a year, you [] your teenager, if you think she's capable of hearing it without be[ing] alarmed about it, that you might have gained that annual pound by eati[ng] 10 calories over your caloric expenditure a day: 10 calories × 365 days/y[ear] 3,650 calories, or about 1 pound of body fat.)

• With all of the diets out there that promote different food combi[na]tions or restrictions of fats or carbohydrates, the bottom line is how the cal[o]ric intake–expenditure equation is modified. This is what ultimately deter[]mines weight balance. Some foods need a bit more energy to digest than others, so energy expenditure is slightly modified by the types of foods you eat. But the main way to change the balance is to change the numbers of calories consumed or the amount expended in physical activity.

• This is why it's helpful to have a sense of the caloric content of foods and of the caloric expenditure of the activities we do. It can be helpful to know that a gram of fat has nine calories and that a gram of protein or carbohydrate has only four calories. This means that fat added to food, such as mayonnaise in sandwiches, butter on potatoes, and cream sauces with pasta, will greatly increase its caloric content.

It can also be helpful to know a bit about the caloric values of the serving sizes of foods, for example, to know that a thin slice of bread (such as a standard slice of Wonder Bread) has about 70 calories and that a large bagel is equivalent to 3–4 slices of bread and thus has about 210–280 calories, in making a choice. Or that a teaspoon of butter or oil has about 45 calories (9 calories × 5 grams of fat), in deciding how much spread to put on your bread or dressing on your salad. Or that soda pop has a lot of empty calories. (Did you know that a 6.5-ounce serving of soda pop—remember those cute little bottles?—has 78 calories, whereas a 64-ounce serving, as in the 7-Eleven Double Gulp, has nearly 10 times that amount—about 750 calories?)

• It can be helpful to know that the meatball sub at Subway has more calories than the veggie delight sub and that if you get the 12-inch instead of the 6-inch, you'll get twice as many calories. But you don't need to know that the 6-inch Veggie Delight sandwich has 232 calories and a Super Meatball 6-inch sub has 594 calories. If your teen knows that much, she is taking things too far. I've been doing this stuff for a long time—and I had to look those numbers up.

Sound familiar? Most of us know better than to tell our children that they need to eat everything on their plates "because there are starving children in the world," but I don't know many parents who haven't struggled with the issue of portion sizes with their kids at some point. What do I do if my kids eat too much? Want dessert but haven't finished the main course? Refuse to try foods or eat too little?

We talked about calorie counting first in this chapter because it is so central to unhealthy weight control measures and disordered eating among teenagers. Although the balance between energy intake and expenditure is what ultimately determines whether one loses, maintains, or gains weight, too much focus on counting calories can backfire and be harmful for your teen. An alternative to calorie counting is portion control. Portion control is a critical issue for all of us, for two reasons:

1. We're all being encouraged to eat bigger meals and snacks than ever before—and usually more than we need.
2. We need to have some way to determine how much is about the right amount of food to eat for our energy expenditure.

Keeping an eye on portion size—without getting obsessed about it—is a good alternative to counting calories.

WHAT YOU'RE UP AGAINST: A TREND TOWARD HUGE PORTIONS

Whether at a restaurant or at home, research has shown that portion sizes have increased considerably over the years, which means that kids may need help in determining what a "normal" portion size really is. Two studies that examined the trends over the last few decades are described on the following page.

Since a daily increase of only 10 calories can lead to a weight gain of one pound in a year, findings from both of these studies suggest that portion sizes may have contributed to the increase in the prevalence of obesity that occurred during the same period. Their findings certainly indicate why paying attention to portion sizes is so important to healthy weight management and overall health promotion. Isn't it interesting that portion sizes have increased in the home as well as in restaurants? Obviously, our sense of what a portion size should be has been distorted by what is available elsewhere. Or perhaps we need larger portions because we're expending so much energy searching for our cordless phones and remote controls.

PORTION SIZE ON THE RISE

Drs. Lisa Young and Marion Nestle found:

- From 1970 to 1999, there was a huge increase in the number of large-size portions introduced, as indicated in the diagram on the facing page.
- New editions of classic cookbooks claim that recipes producing the same amount of food as in the original edition serve fewer people.
- Auto manufacturers have installed larger cup holders in newer models.
- Restaurants are using larger dinner plates, bakers are using larger muffin tins, pizzerias are using larger pans, and fast-food companies are using larger drink and french fry containers.
- Food companies now use larger sizes as selling points; fast-food restaurants promote larger items with signs, place mats, and staff pins; and manufacturers of diet meals advertise larger meal sizes.
- All food portions measured, with the exception of a slice of white bread, exceeded serving sizes described in the food guide pyramid.

Drs. Samara Nielsen and Barry Popkin found the following trends at home, in fast-food outlets, and at other restaurants in 1977–1998:

- Portion sizes increased for most categories of food, at home and away.
- The average portion size of salty snack foods increased from 1.0 to 1.6 ounces, by 93 calories.
- The average portion size of soft drinks increased from 13.1 to 19.9 fluid ounces, by 49 calories.
- Hamburger size increased from 5.7 to 7.0 ounces, by 97 calories.
- An average portion of french fries increased from 3.1 to 3.6 ounces, by 68 calories.
- An average portion of Mexican food increased from 6.3 to 8.0 ounces, by 133 calories.
- Portion sizes for most foods were largest at fast-food restaurants, including salty snacks, soft drinks, fruit drinks, french fries, and Mexican food.
- For desserts, hamburgers, and cheeseburgers, the largest portion sizes were found at home.

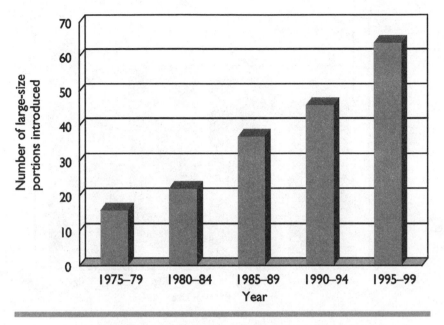

Increasing numbers of large portion sizes.

From Young LR, Nestle, M. The contribution of expanding portion sizes to the US obesity epidemic. *American Journal of Public Health.* 2002; **92**: 246–249. Copyright 2002 by the American Public Health Association. Reprinted by permission.

JUST BECAUSE THERE'S MORE FOOD ON MY PLATE DOESN'T MEAN I'M GOING TO EAT IT ALL ... OR DOES IT?

In a series of studies, Dr. Barbara Rolls and her colleagues found a clear answer in older children and adults: Getting larger portions *does* translate to eating larger portions. As shown in the diagram on the next page, study participants who were served 1,000 grams of macaroni and cheese ate more than those served 500 grams; they consumed 162 calories more. Similar results were found with other foods such as sandwiches and potato chips. Interestingly, members of both groups reported feeling full—and those who ate the larger portions did not seem to compensate by eating less at later meals or during the next day. *Most interesting of all, very young children were not affected by portion size; apparently they eat according to internal signs of hunger and satiety.* By the age of five, however, the amount of food eaten was affected by portion size. Somewhere along the way, our children learn to pay less attention to internal signs of hunger and more attention to external stimuli to eat. This finding hints at the most important methods for regulating how much we eat.

Portion Control and Calorie Counting

163

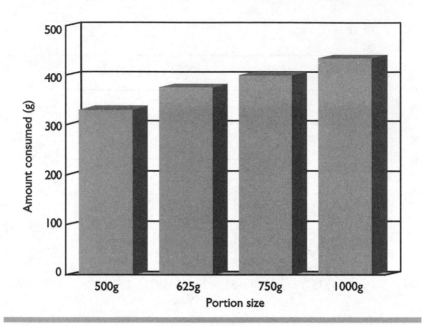

Macaroni and cheese intake by portion size in adults.

From Rolls BJ, Morris EI, Roe LA. Portion size of food affects energy intake in normal-weight and overweight men and women. *American Journal of Clinical Nutrition.* 2002; **76:** 1207–1213. Copyright 2002 by the American Society for Clinical Nutrition. Adapted by permission. As adapted in Rolls BJ. The supersizing of America: Portion size and the obesity epidemic. *Nutrition Today.* 2003; **38**(2): 42–53. Reprinted by permission of Lippincott Williams & Wilkins.

What You Can Do to Help Your Teen Eat Reasonably Sized Portions

1. FIND OUT WHY YOUR TEENAGER IS OVEREATING (OR UNDEREATING)

• **Does your child lack knowledge about the caloric content of foods?** Offer the short course provided in the list on pages 158–160, making sure the overall discussion centers on behavior, not weight, and doesn't make your child feel bad about herself.

• **Is your teen experiencing some kind of emotional turmoil?** Has something happened that your teen is trying to forget about? Has your teen been the victim of weight teasing? Might your teen be numbing or "stuffing" emotions? Does your teen have some emotional needs that are not being met? Take time to explore these issues with your teen, and consider talking with a psychologist if there seems to be an underlying disturbance.

- **Does your teen suffer from depression? Loneliness? Low self-esteem? Boredom?** If so, talking about portion sizes and calories won't solve the underlying problem . . . and might make it worse. Again, try to spend some extra time with your teen and think about external resources that might be helpful, such as professional help or a different social group.

- **What do meals look like in your family?** Does your family eat out a lot? Bring home food from fast-food outlets? Do you eat as a family? Is a lot of food served? What kinds of food? Is there tension at meals? Take some time to explore what you can do to change family meal practices to make them more conducive to healthy food choices. We will look in more depth at family meal and family eating-out practices in the next section (Chapters 11–13).

- **Does your teen come home from school or come to meals hungry as a result of not eating enough throughout the day?** This is a frequent cause of overeating, particularly among teens who are trying to "save on calories." Talk about how skipping meals tends to backfire and do what you can to help your teen eat something before leaving for school in the morning.

- **Are your children eating large portions because of their fear of being hungry later on and not being allowed to eat?** Sometimes parents impose rules about when kids can eat when they're trying to help their children control their food intake. If this sounds familiar, make sure your children know that when they get hungry they can eat again . . . and won't have to "sneak."

- **Is eating large portions the norm in your house?** If you typically serve large portions and family members typically overeat when good food is around or in response to stress, consider how you can change your home environment to make it easier for your teenager to eat appropriate portion sizes.

2. STRESS THE IDEA THAT YOUR KIDS SHOULD EAT WHEN HUNGRY AND STOP WHEN FULL

Our bodies are designed to send us signals of hunger when we need fuel. And as the study done by Rolls and colleagues, mentioned earlier, shows, until age five this "fuel gauge" seems to work pretty well. Very young children eat when they're hungry and stop when they're full. After age five, however, we're apparently stimulated to eat just by what's available in front of us. So it's critical to help our children to keep associating eating with feelings of hunger as they enter adolescence—in a way that's sensitive to their feelings.

I look for opportunities to reinforce eating (or not eating) according to hunger level whenever possible. When my kids say they're not hungry, I'll say something like "It's good that you're paying attention to what your body is telling you." If they make comments such as "I can't believe I ate so much, I'll say something like "Well, you were probably hungry after being at the beach all day." As in most cases, looking for opportunities to reinforce desirable behaviors, rather than pointing out or commenting on undesirable behaviors, is always preferable.

---

what you can do
THINK BEFORE YOU SPEAK

Before making a comment on your teen's eating behaviors, think about how it may affect your relationship and further communication on food- and weight-related topics. Is it worth the risk? Even if you're trying to reinforce the hunger–eating connection, commenting in any way on how much food your teen is eating, especially within earshot of others, can have an unwanted effect. Unless you're positive that the comment won't be read as a criticism, consider saying nothing. If there's information you really want to impart, save it for later when it won't be connected to the teen's behavior at all.

Of course, there is a caveat to all this. When you try to explain the concept of relying on hunger to your teenagers, say that while a comfortable amount of hunger is a sign that they should eat, they should try to avoid getting too hungry since that sets them up for binge eating or consuming large portions without giving enough thought to what they are eating. Furthermore, Dr. Moria Golan, who runs an eating disorder clinic in Israel, warns that kids who say they aren't hungry all day, are repeatedly not hungry at meals, or are hungry all day long, have lost the connection between hunger and eating and require intervention (see Chapter 15).

It's essential for our children to learn to pay attention to their own bodies and what these physiological signals tell them with regard to being full or wanting to eat more. That doesn't mean that parents don't have a role to play here, even with teenagers. As discussed throughout this book, parents can do much by providing a home environment that is conducive to appropriate portion sizes and serving as role models by eating appropriate amounts of food. *But the general rule should be to let your kids make the final decision about how much to eat. Trying to control how much they eat is likely to be counterproductive.*

DIVIDING RESPONSIBILITIES FOR PORTION CONTROL

Ellyn Satter writes that it's the parent's role to provide healthy food within a healthy atmosphere, but it's the child's role to decide how much to eat, since this will help the child develop good internal regulation regarding eating patterns and recognizing satiety. She says parents are responsible for *what, when,* and *where,* and children are responsible for *how much* and *whether.* This means it's your job to decide what to prepare, when food is to be eaten or meals are to be served, and where they are to be eaten. The child makes the decision about whether to eat what is being served and how much to eat. Although her writing focuses mainly on younger children, Satter's advice is also relevant for teenagers (with a bit more flexibility of course). Her words of wisdom have the potential to prevent many struggles over food at the dinner table and the development of a range of eating problems. (See *www.ellynsatter.com* for more helpful hints.)

3. MODEL APPROPRIATE PORTION SIZES

Do you overeat at restaurants, or after a stressful day, or in response to negative emotions? Do you avoid eating during the day and overeat at night? What do your own portion sizes look like? Do you count calories? Talk about calories? Take time to explore your own behaviors and think about gradual changes you're ready to make. When you go out to eat with your kids, split large entrées, bring doggie bags home, and avoid the supersize specials. If you eat excessively after a stressful day, look for alternative healthier behaviors. You can have a large impact on your children's portion sizes without saying a word.

4. MAKE SMALL CHANGES IN THE WAYS YOU PROVIDE AND SERVE FOOD

Take a look at the following ideas and choose one that works for your family:

- If your teens are responsible for grabbing their own meals and snacks more often than not, provide a bit more structure by preparing a meal when you can.
- Purchase portioned foods instead of jumbo bags of chips and bakery items.
- Help your kids learn to choose an appropriate portion by letting them

serve themselves, but avoid putting out heaps of food; they should understand that what's on the table has to feed everyone. (If you prepare food for more than one meal, don't put it all out on the table.)

• If you prefer to serve the food yourself, serve small first helpings. When you offer seconds, ask, "Is anyone still hungry?" rather than just, "Would anyone like some more?"

• The idea of saving room for dessert may actually help children and teens feel they don't need to take a second serving. Try it out in your home, and include some healthy dessert options such as fresh fruit, fruit salad, canned fruit, or sorbet; or portioned foods like cookies, cups of pudding, ice cream bars, or miniature candy bars.

• If eating a lot of food very quickly is a problem at your house, serve some foods that take a bit longer to eat—foods that require chewing such as raw vegetables and salads and foods with higher water content such as soup. Bulk and high nutrient density can also help with big appetites. Foods such as soup, salad, and cut-up vegetables are often packed with nutrients, so your teens will get what they need from what they eat; they are also "bulky" foods that take a fair amount of time to consume in relation to the amount of calories they contain. I'm sure you've seen a teenage boy eat a hamburger in about 30 seconds, a feat that's just not possible with a big bowl of salad filled with crunchy veggies or a hearty, steaming bowl of soup. There may be some truth in the belief that "it takes 20 minutes for the brain to register what's gone into the stomach." In any event, it is certainly true that if you are through eating before anyone else at the table, you aren't just going to want to sit there watching everyone else eat.

what you can do
TALK ABOUT PORTION AND CREATIVE PORTION CONTROL

When you see an opportunity, and your teen isn't in the midst of biting into a humongous sandwich, talk about how disproportionate the large servings are in restaurants, fast-food outlets, and movie theaters. Compare portion sizes commonly served in restaurants with portion sizes served in an airplane meal. Although airplane portions may seem small, they are actually more in line with the portion sizes that most of us should be eating.

Also let your teens know that there are two ways to aim for portion control. One way is by eating smaller portion sizes: Order the small instead of the large; share entrées; avoid buying supersize bags of chips, and so forth. The other way is to think about food *content*. By eating foods that are low in calories but high in volume because of a high water content (such as fruits, vegetables, salads, and soups), you can feel full and satisfied. You'll eat fewer calories even though your portion is large.

What's a Parent to Do?

At the beginning of this chapter I said that when it comes to how much to eat, there's no getting around making specific decisions in the moment. So I'm going to put my money where my mouth is and make some recommendations for the parents of Gary, Liora, Sophie, and Stuart (with the understanding that optimal decisions will depend on more information, such as the nature of the relationships between these teens and their parents, their weight-related concerns, and their sensitivity to discussing eating behaviors). If you've read this chapter, you might already have the same ideas.

With regard to Gary and Stuart, if they were my children, I would probably hold off on commenting about their portion sizes at the fast-food restaurant or at the movies and talk about portion sizes at another time, without referring to their behaviors. For example, I might make a comment about an article that I was reading about fast-food supersizing. Depending on the situation, I might ask if they want to split an order with me. I would definitely take a look at the kind of role modeling we do in our family: For example, when we go out to eat, do we ever share large entrées?

With regard to Liora, her mother has made the right decision not to ask about the calories in the foods she wants to order. But the fact that Liora has a calorie counter in her purse and is using it to guide her food selection has me concerned. If there has been a change in Liora's behaviors, her mother should explore the possible reasons for this change. She should talk with her daughter about the negatives of calorie counting and present some alternatives such as portion control and food choices guided by the food guide pyramid and by internal cues of hunger and satiety. I would encourage Liora's mother to examine her own calorie counting and other weight-related behaviors.

I would recommend that Sophie's mother not comment on Sophie's taking a second helping of spaghetti at dinner. Any such remark is bound to create hard feelings that will be either stored inside or shared at the table and lead to an argument. First of all, it's possible that Sophie needs a second helping if she's had an active day. But if it really does seem as though Sophie's energy intake exceeds her expenditure, her parents might want to explore why she is so hungry at dinner (did she skip lunch or miss an after-school snack?). To avoid this behavior on the future, they might serve soup before the main course and a salad with the spaghetti, put less food on the table to encourage everyone to take appropriate serving sizes, and try to get in the habit of serving a healthful dessert, such as fruit, so that everyone knows something else is coming.

10

Vegetarianism
Doing It Right—for Your Teen and Your Family

*J*essica is a competitive runner. She watches what she eats and tries to keep her weight down, since she believes this helps her speed. One night at dinner, when her mother passes around the chicken, Jessica says, "No thanks. I've decided to become a vegetarian." Her mother isn't quite sure how to respond and wonders if Jessica is just trying to legitimize the exclusion of additional foods from her diet.

Since Paul started middle school, he has been pulling away from his family in different ways. His family tends to be meat and potato eaters; thus, his parents are not at all happy when Paul decides to become a vegetarian. His father feels that Paul is rejecting their family's way of eating. Paul's mother is concerned about the adequacy of Paul's diet, since he is excluding all kinds of foods without adding nutritionally equivalent substitutes. She also misses having Paul at family meals; he says there's really not much point in joining the family because they're eating foods that he can't eat and just seeing meat on the table bothers him.

Shayna's family has always consumed a lot of plant-based foods, so when Shayna became a vegetarian a few years ago, it wasn't a surprise to her family, nor did it make meal planning particularly burdensome. However, when she returned home from college for summer break, she told her parents that she had decided to become a vegan and eliminate dairy foods and eggs from her diet. This has her parents concerned about her motivation for these additional restrictions and about the nutritional adequacy of her intake.

As you've already read, obesity is increasingly rapidly among teenagers. A third of our teenagers are overweight or at risk of becoming overweight. About half of our teens eat more fat than recommended. More than two-thirds are eating less than the recommended three to five servings a day of fruits and vegetables. And even more teens are eating inadequate amounts of deep green or yellow vegetables, whole grain products, and legumes.

So you might be surprised to hear that a red flag goes up for me when a teenager says he's decided to become a vegetarian. I'll sound the clarion call for kids to eat a lot more fruits and veggies till I'm blue (or green) in the face. But as you'll read in this chapter, I believe we should exercise caution when our kids announce that they want to cut animal products out of their daily diet—for nutritional as well as psychological reasons. (Everything in this chapter, incidentally, is based on the assumption that your family is *not* currently following a vegetarian diet. If you are, then your teenager's desire to be a vegetarian may not have the same psychological implications, and you probably already know how to satisfy everyone's nutritional needs.)

For parents of the kids described at the beginning of this chapter, the key to determining how to respond is to find out what the teenager means by *vegetarian* and why he or she wants to make this change.

What Does Your Teenager Mean by *Vegetarian*?

Vegetarianism means eliminating certain foods from the diet, which may require substituting others to ensure adequate nutrition. So it's important to know what your teenager has in mind. In Project EAT, 6% of the teens (193 girls and 69 boys) said they were vegetarians, but, as the table on the facing page shows, most of them were not strict vegetarians.

Although it seems a bit strange that so many of the "vegetarians" in this study were actually "semi-vegetarians," other studies have found the same thing. In a study of young women in college, 77% of the 30 students who claimed to be vegetarians ate either fish or chicken. It's hard to say whether cutting out red meat is simply what most young people mean by vegetarian-

DIFFERENT TYPES OF VEGETARIAN EATING PATTERNS AND PREVALENCE AMONG 262 TEENS WHO REPORTED BEING VEGETARIANS IN PROJECT EAT

Type	Food exclusions	% of vegetarians
Vegan	Excludes all foods of animal origin: dairy food, eggs, meat, poultry, and fish.	6%
Ovo-vegetarian	Excludes meat, poultry, fish, and dairy foods. Includes eggs.	2%
Lacto-vegetarian	Excludes eggs, meat, poultry, and fish. Includes dairy foods.	11%
Lacto-ovo vegetarian	Excludes meat, poultry, and fish. Includes eggs and dairy foods.	21%
Semi-vegetarian	Usually excludes red meat, but may include small amounts of fish or poultry.	60%

ism or whether that's just the first step taken by many of those desiring a vegetarian lifestyle. Interestingly, the gradations of vegetarianism adopted have disparate implications, and some of them might surprise you.

For example, as far as nutrition is concerned, vegan and ovo-vegetarian diets, because they omit eggs and dairy foods or just dairy foods, respectively, pose the greatest challenges for meeting a teenager's dietary needs. That's somewhat obvious. It also may be somewhat obvious that the vegetarians who omit all animal-based foods are those who are motivated mainly by a desire to avoid killing animals. But you might also think that the greater the restrictions, the more interested the teens would be in adopting this diet to manage their weight. Not so. Project EAT found that 48% of semi-vegetarians were motivated by an interest in weight control, as compared with only 28% of the more restrictive vegetarians.

For vegans, your main concern as a parent might be the specter of nutritional deficiencies, particularly in regard to calcium and vitamin B_{12}, both of which come largely from animal products. For semi-vegetarians, the biggest issue might be that a focus on weight control carries the risk of eating disorders down the road.

To many teenagers, especially younger ones, *vegetarian* just sounds like a noble thing to be, either for vague animal-protection and environmental reasons or because it seems like a healthy choice. Ask what your teen has in mind.

Does she intend to cut out just red meat, or poultry and fish too? Will she be eating milk products and eggs? Does she know the various terms to designate these variations of vegetarianism and what they mean? Does she fully understand what choices these restrictions might leave her with? (In a hilarious talk show a number of years ago, the guest was a young woman who professed to be a total vegetarian " . . . except for, like, burgers, man.") If you have a young teenager, he may very well not have thought this through, and it will help him crystallize his intentions if you talk it out.

Your teen may also not understand what must be added to her diet if she cuts out certain foods in the name of vegetarianism. Becoming a vegetarian should not simply mean cutting out certain foods, rather teens need to think about the foods they will be adding to their diets. In Israel, where I used to live, falafel, hummus, tahini, nuts, and seeds are cheap and sold everywhere on the street, but in the United States teens may have to make a much bigger effort to find easy alternatives to meat.

what you can do
HELP YOUR TEEN FIND VEGETARIAN FAST FOOD

There are great alternatives to the typical fast-food chains, though they might not be quite as fast to pick up. Neighborhood Mediterranean restaurants often have falafel and hummus and the like to go. The little Asian restaurants—even the chains—have vegetarian options that substitute tofu for meat, use lots of dark green leafy vegetables, and often make brown rice available instead of white. Finally, a growing trend toward "new" Mexican chains makes some delicious bean-based vegetarian options available, with lots of veggies part of every offering. Many teens end up liking these highly flavored foods more than their previous favorite burgers and fries.

what you can do
DON'T LOSE THIS OPPORTUNITY TO GET YOUR TEEN INTERESTED IN NUTRITION

Expressions of interest in vegetarianism are your cue to get your teen interested in nutrition. I remember reading, as a teen, *Diet for a Small Planet* (by F. M. Lappe) with great fervor. I have included some teen-friendly resources on nutrition at the end of this book; I suggest purchasing a book or two, going to the library and seeing what is available there, and taking a look on the Internet. Websites that you and your teen might find useful include *www.vrg.org* (an excellent resource offered by the Vegetarian Resource Group), *www. vegsoc.org* (a lot of great information from the Vegetarian Society of the United Kingdom, including a booklet for parents and teens that can be downloaded free of charge), (*www.vegetariantimes.com*) (great recipes), and *www.nlm.nih.gov/medlineplus/vegetarianism.html* (includes a number of links to other sites and can be a useful resource for you). This can be a wonderful opportunity for expanding your teen's interest in nutrition beyond that of weight control—and for showing your teenager that you care.

DOES YOUR TEEN KNOW
WHAT HEALTHY VEGETARIANISM INVOLVES?

A number of food guides have been developed for vegetarian diets. In general, these guides promote the following:

- The intake of meat alternatives such as legumes (chickpeas, beans, and lentils), soy products (soybeans, soy milk, tofu, and tempeh), nuts, and seeds.
- The importance of mixing proteins to complement incomplete proteins found in many plant-based foods. Your teen will need to eat legumes with grains (beans and rice), legumes with seeds (falafel with tahini sauce), and grains with milk (milk and cereal). Research has suggested that this mixing can be done over the course of a few hours or a day and that complementary proteins do not need to be eaten at the same time.
- The intake of alternatives to dairy products for vegans and ovo-vegetarians. Most important, food guides have addressed the need for adequate calcium intake and how to look for foods that are good sources of absorbable calcium among the different food groups (for example, orange juice, breakfast cereal, and soy milk that have been fortified with calcium.
- The importance of ensuring adequate intake of B_{12} and vitamin D in vegans, usually through supplements or fortified foods and adequate sun exposure (for vitamin D).

The food guide pyramid introduced in Chapter 8 can be helpful to vegetarians as well as omnivores, as long as vegetarians (1) substitute protein alternatives for meats and (2) add sources of calcium-rich foods if they are vegans. When you talk to your teen about what she has in mind, have the food pyramid handy to help you think and plan.

Vegetarianism

175

Why Does Your Teenager Want to Become a Vegetarian?

This is a critical question, because it can inform you about the wisdom of this decision for your individual adolescent. The next table shows that in Project EAT, *the most commonly reported reason for becoming a vegetarian was to lose weight or keep from gaining weight;* a third of the vegetarians reported doing so for weight management purposes. Approximately one-fourth of the vegetarians cited not wanting to kill animals, not liking the taste of meat, or wanting a healthier diet.

WHAT ARE YOUR MAIN REASONS FOR EATING A VEGETARIAN DIET?

To lose weight or keep from gaining weight	35%
Do not want to kill animals	28%
I don't like the taste of meat	27%
Want a healthier diet	25%
To help the environment	17%
A family member is a vegetarian	14%
Religious reasons	10%

Responses from 262 self-reported teenage vegetarians in Project EAT. Since teens could record more than one reason, percentages do not add up to 100%. The data are from Perry CL, McGuire MT, Neumark-Sztainer D, Story M. Characteristics of vegetarian adolescents in a multiethnic urban population. *Journal of Adolescent Health.* 2001; 29: 406–416.

what you can do
HELP YOUR TEENAGER UNDERSTAND THAT A VEGETARIAN DIET IS NOT NECESSARILY A BETTER WEIGHT MANAGEMENT STRATEGY THAN A NONVEGETARIAN DIET

A vegetarian diet can be helpful in reducing total fat and saturated fat intake if high-fat meats are replaced with soy products, other legumes, and whole grains. But refer your teen to Chapter 9 and remind her about balancing energy intake with energy expenditure. Also let your teen know that a vegetarian diet is not necessarily lower in calories than a nonvegetarian diet. A huge heap of rice or pasta, a cup of nuts or seeds, or a serving of tortilla chips with guacamole can have more calories than a three-ounce portion of chicken or red meat. And vegetarians who eliminate meat but include foods like Cinnabons, Mrs. Field's cookies, and Cheetos in their daily diets, and wash them down with Mountain Dew, obviously won't be shedding pounds.

THE PROS AND CONS OF VEGETARIANISM
FOR WEIGHT CONTROL

The Pros

• Adult vegetarians tend to be less overweight and to have fewer obesity-related health problems. Research has shown that adult vegetarians have lower body weight in relation to their height (body mass index, or BMI) than nonvegetarians, tend to live longer, and have lower rates of cardiovascular diseases, hypertension (high blood pressure), Type 2 diabetes, and some types of cancer. These health benefits are, at least in part, probably due to healthier lifestyles above and beyond their dietary intake. For example, they may smoke less and be more physically active. However, there are substantial differences in dietary intake between adult vegetarians and nonvegetarians that clearly also contribute to these health benefits.

• In our own work, we have *not* found differences in body mass index or obesity prevalence between vegetarian and nonvegetarian teens, and this is a significant factor you should take into account when talking about the weight control benefits of vegetarianism with your son or daughter. However, vegetarian teens are more likely to eat in accordance with dietary recommendations. In Project EAT, 70% of the vegetarians got less than 30% of their calories from fat, as compared with only 45% of the nonvegetarians; 65% of the vegetarians got less than 10% of their calories from saturated fat, as compared with 39% of the nonvegetarians; and 39% of the vegetarians ate five or more daily servings of fruits and vegetables, as compared with 28% of the nonvegetarians. Teen vegetarians also ate less fast food and drank less soda pop and fruit drinks. Another study, using data from the Minnesota Adolescent Health Survey, found that vegetarian teens were twice as likely to eat fruits and vegetables as nonvegetarian teens, one-third as likely to eat sweets, and one-fourth as likely to eat salty snack foods more than once a day.

• The dietary intakes of the teen vegetarians and the lower rates of obesity among the adult vegetarians suggest that if teens continue to eat a plant-based diet, they may be less likely to be overweight as adults.

• In Project EAT, teenage vegetarians cared more about eating healthy food and felt more confident in their ability to make healthy food choices in different settings.

• A vegetarian diet has advantages for the environment. The foods vegetarians eat are lower on the food chain. Lesser amounts of the earth's resources are used to grow vegetables and grain than to raise animals for meat.

We can feed more people on earth with plant-based diets than with animal-based diets.

- A vegetarian diet is definitely beneficial for animals. A plant-based diet for more people would prevent fewer animals from being raised in conditions that are ideal for food production, but not ideal for the animals or the workers who help to raise them.

The Cons

- Research suggests that some teens may become vegetarians as a socially acceptable way to eliminate certain foods from their diets, particularly foods that tend to have a higher fat content. Peter, a high school teen, used the excuse of being a vegetarian to avoid eating the spaghetti and meatballs his family served for dinner, diverting them from objecting when he said he'd just have the salad and broccoli.

- In Project EAT, we found that vegetarian teens were much more likely to display an unhealthy preoccupation with weight, unhealthy weight control behaviors, disordered eating, and eating disorders, than nonvegetarian teens. Three times as many vegetarians report that a doctor had told them that they had an eating disorder such as anorexia nervosa, bulimia nervosa, or binge eating disorder, as shown in the following table.

- Interestingly, vegetarian boys were just as likely as vegetarian girls to weigh themselves often and engage in unhealthy weight control behaviors.

WEIGHT-RELATED PROBLEMS IN VEGETARIAN AND NONVEGETARIAN TEENS

	Vegetarians	Nonvegetarians
"I weigh myself often"	40%	31%
Used unhealthy weight control behaviors in last year	69%	44%
Vomited in past week for weight control	9%	3%
Used diet pills in past week	6%	2%
Used laxatives in past week for weight control	6%	1%
Were told by doctor that they have an eating disorder	9%	3%

The data are from Perry CL, McGuire MT, Neumark-Sztainer D, Story M. Characteristics of vegetarian adolescents in a multiethnic urban population. *Journal of Adolescent Health*. 2001; 29: 406–416.

Usually, these behaviors are much lower in boys than in girls. This indicates that *although being a vegetarian can be a red flag for weight-related problems in girls, it is even more indicative in boys.* Adopting a vegetarian diet may be more socially acceptable for boys interested in weight loss than a more typical weight loss diet, which may be viewed as a "girl's thing." If your son is a vegetarian, does that mean he has an eating disorder? Absolutely not. But it can serve to remind you to keep a slightly closer watch on what he is eating and to take a bit more time to talk with him about what's going on in his life.

- Other studies have also found that vegetarians may be at risk for disordered eating. Among middle school and high school teens who participated in the Minnesota Adolescent Health Survey, we found that vegetarians were almost twice as likely to diet frequently, four times as likely to make themselves vomit for weight control purposes, and eight times as likely to use laxatives for weight control, as nonvegetarians. Among young women in college, 37% of vegetarians were at risk for eating disorders as compared with 8% of the nonvegetarians. The vegetarians were more likely to report attitudes and behaviors such as being preoccupied with a desire to be thinner, exercising strenuously to burn off calories, feeling that food controls their lives, and having the impulse to vomit after meals. In a study of a clinical population of 116 patients with anorexia nervosa, 54% of the patients were avoiding red meat, which was associated with a longer duration of anorexia nervosa.

In Balance

So, adopting a vegetarian eating style may provide teens with a legitimate and effective means of weight management as long as they can incorporate healthy eating patterns into their lifestyle and, for example, replace high-fat meats with lower-fat legumes. But for teens who aren't concerned with the nutritional adequacy of their food intake or for those who are developing disordered eating, adopting a vegetarian diet often provides a way to disguise a problem.

As mentioned earlier, it's ironic that the red flag may be waving more urgently for semi-vegetarian teens than for more restrictive vegetarians. In our study, 75% of the semi-vegetarians reported unhealthy weight control behaviors, as compared with 57% of the more restrictive vegetarians. We also found that semi-vegetarians were less likely to be eating according to the dietary guidelines than more restrictive vegetarians; semi-vegetarians ate fewer fruits and vegetables, and more of their calories came from fat.

For some of these teens, trying to become a vegetarian may just be another way of trying to control their weight. Semi-vegetarians may still be in a

RESEARCH SHOWS NO DIRECT CAUSE-AND-EFFECT RELATIONSHIP BETWEEN VEGETARIANISM AND EATING DISORDERS

I am often asked, "Does vegetarianism lead to eating disorders?" In a small proportion of cases, teens may start off with a vegetarian diet, enjoy taking control and having certain restrictions on what they eat, lose weight, get compliments, go too far, and go on to develop an eating disorder. But this is the exception rather than the rule.

I believe that in most cases the sequence of events is reversed and teens who are already on their way to developing disordered eating behaviors may adopt vegetarianism as an additional strategy for restricting food intake. So, the answer is that vegetarianism is unlikely to cause an eating disorder, but it may be a sign of an emerging problem, alerting parents to pay attention to what else may be going on with their teen.

stage of transition from a meat-based diet to a plant-based diet; they may not have the same ideology that more restrictive vegetarians have; and they may not be putting the same thought into planning their dietary intake.

what you can do

IF YOUR TEENAGER DOESN'T TAKE YOUR INPUT SERIOUSLY, FIND OTHER RESOURCES TO HELP HIM OR HER MAKE AN INFORMED DECISION

There are tons of teen friendly books on vegetarianism, vegetarian magazines, and Internet sources for reliable information. Most general nutrition books for teens also include a section on vegetarianism. A few are listed at the back of this book. If things get a bit tense, arrange to meet with a dietitian who has experience in working with teens.

Take-Home Message

If you have a teen who has decided to "become a vegetarian," explore your teen's motivations for doing so and get some teen-friendly resources on planning a vegetarian diet in a way that ensures nutritional adequacy. Do this even, or especially, if your teen is a semi-vegetarian. Also, think carefully about your teen's risk for weight-related problems. Go back to Chapter 2 and look at the spheres of influence on weight-related issues, asking yourself the questions about your teenager in the worksheet in that chapter. Does your teen have body image concerns? Does your teen diet? Has your teen recently lost weight? Have you noticed a recent change in your teen's eating patterns, such as not wanting to join the family for meals or being picky about food choices? Do your teen's friends engage in fat talk? In your family, is there a lot of talk about weight? Is your teen involved in sports in which weight is a big issue? Has your teen been the victim of weight teasing?

If you answered "no" to these questions, then your teen's adoption of a vegetarian diet may be part of his search for identity as a teenager. Ask him about his reasons and show respect for his reasons, whether they include concern for animal welfare, environmental preservation, or overall health. It will be important for you to show your support, work out the logistics with your teen (see the following section), and help him attain a nutritionally balanced dietary intake. However, his interest in vegetarianism is very unlikely to be a sign of an emerging eating disorder.

If you answered "yes" to more than one of these questions, then becoming a vegetarian may be another strategy for your teen to restrict food intake. Take some time to explore what is going on in your teen's life and offer your support. Pay a bit more attention to what your teen is eating and, without overreacting, make more of an effort to make eating easier for your teen by having more regular family meals. If you feel as though you're being manipulated, don't be afraid to be firm about what you're willing to do to help your teen and what it's okay for your teen to do.

How to Adapt If Your Teenager Decides to Adopt a Vegetarian Diet

If the rest of your family does not follow a vegetarian diet, you'll need to discuss your expectations with your teen, and everyone (definitely including the vegetarian teen) will have to be willing to make compromises and help out. An up-front discussion aimed at helping your teen, while sharing the workload, can go a long way.

| what you can do CLARIFY EXPECTATIONS AND COME UP WITH A GAME PLAN IN ADVANCE | Make this planning a condition of your teen's starting on this new eating plan. Sit down together after you've gathered whatever resources you need—cookbooks, information |

on vegetarian nutrition, grocery lists, and so forth. Talk with your teen about alternative foods that he will be including in his diet in place of those he will be excluding. Figure out what will work best for your family and who will do what. How old is your teenager, and how capable of participating in food preparation? What's negotiable here? Remind your teenager that others in the family have their own nutritional and other needs, from the young kids who need lots of calcium, which comes most easily from dairy products, to others in the family who need a low intake of fat and should therefore not center meals on cheese instead of chicken. Some meals can be vegetarian for everyone, but for others . . . your teen can make himself a veggie burger.

DON'T CHANGE EVERYTHING

Don't change everything because of your teen. By the time you have made substantial changes in planning meals, your teen may have turned back into a steak lover. But I think three things are important here:

1. **Show you're interested in helping your teen.** Can you make a couple of vegetarian meals a week? Can you stock up on some vegetarian foods that will make things easy for your teen? Can the two of you come up with a list of favorite family meals that can be served both with and without meat without a lot of extra trouble? Spaghetti and marinara sauce, with the meatballs in a separate bowl? Tacos or burritos that everyone fills for him- or herself, with bowls full of veggies, cheese, and other such items, and a separate bowl for chicken or meat?

2. **Make it clear that your teen still needs to come to family meals.** Your teen still needs to be present at family meals. On days when you aren't having vegetarian foods, your teen can make something easy for himself to eat or can eat the side dishes and have a glass of milk and a peanut butter and jelly sandwich, some pita bread with hummus, or some granola with yogurt.

3. **Don't let all the extra workload fall on you.** Brainstorm some ideas that will work for your family. Can your teen prepare a vegetarian meal once a week and give you a break? Do some of the grocery shopping? Do extra cleanup?

| **what you can do** INSIST ON A DIET FOUNDED IN VARIETY, MODERATION, AND BALANCE | **Variety:** Vegetarian teens need foods from among and within the different food groups. It's particularly important for teens to get variety from within the meat alternative group, since plant- |

based proteins may not be complete on their own.

Moderation: Foods high in fat and sugar should be eaten in moderation, but not totally restricted. Fat intake can be either too low or too high on vegetarian diets; some teens may use their vegetarian diet as a way to totally restrict fat intake, whereas others may assume that because they aren't eating meat, their fat intake will be low.

Balance: Vegetarians need to eat foods in proportion to the sizes of their respective food groups in the food guide pyramid. In many ways this is easier to do on a vegetarian diet, which, if done correctly, will include an abundance of whole grains, fruits, and vegetables, a moderate amount of dairy and meat alternatives, and a sprinkling of extras. Whereas we usually don't worry much about nonvegetarian teens eating enough from the meat group, vegetarian teens will need to make sure they are eating enough legumes, nuts, seeds, tofu, and soy foods. Attention must be paid to getting enough calcium; for teens avoiding dairy products, fortified foods from the different food groups, such as orange juice and breakfast cereals, can be very helpful.

Remember, your teenagers need you to ensure that *adolescent nutrition* is not an oxymoron. They need to eat appropriate portion sizes, to avoid obsessing over counting calories, and to experiment with different eating patterns such as vegetarianism in a way that enhances their nutritional intake. Teens do not develop eating patterns, physical activity behaviors, and weight-related attitudes within a vacuum; rather, they are influenced greatly by family eating patterns, food availability within the home, family norms regarding physical activity, and discussions in the home on matters of food, fitness, and weight. Yet, as parents, we face many more challenges than our parents did in making family meals happen on a regular basis and in discussing sensitive issues regarding food and weight. In the next section (Chapters 11–13) we explore how to establish a healthy home base.

"How can we make
a difference at home . . .
and away?"

11

Family Meals in a Fast-Food World

You probably don't need a research study to tell you that family meals, at which everyone sits down at the table together on a daily basis, are a thing of the past for many of us. But you may have wondered what we're missing by letting this tradition lapse. Because obesity and eating disorders are more prevalent now than they were in the *Leave It to Beaver* and *Father Knows Best* days, as a scientist I wondered too. Of course, I also wondered as a parent—a working parent of teenagers with busy schedules. What *really* goes on in other families? Is it true that everyone eats on the fly these days? What do teenagers think about having breakfast, brunch, lunch, or dinner with the rest of the family? Do we need to stick together for three squares a day to prevent weight-related problems in our kids, or could a few good family meals throughout the week do the trick?

You probably know where I'm going with this: I wanted to know just how guilty I should feel when I needed to work late. I wanted to know how much trouble we'd all have to go through to make changes at our house if it turned out that my instinct was correct—that family meals can help instill healthy eating habits in our kids.

Like you, I did not need a research study to figure out that times have changed, but my colleagues and I dug up some fascinating facts in our studies about exactly how family meals matter, which in turn suggested some not-too-daunting ideas for tweaking the home environment to help our kids develop healthier eating patterns and prevent unhealthy weight control behaviors, binge eating, and possibly an array of other problematic behaviors. This chapter will give you some tips and illustrations for pulling it off.

But before we get into the details, let me make two things perfectly clear:

1. When I say "family meals," what I mean is meals at which family members sit down together and focus their attention on the communal experience of enjoying food—and, we hope, some lively conversation at the same time. I don't mean that the cook has to be Mom or even that all the food has to be home cooked.

2. Family meals prepared from fresh ingredients by the family and eaten at home have some unique benefits to offer aside from nutrition. But that doesn't mean you can't take shortcuts in food preparation or have a family meal at a restaurant; you just have to know the role that restaurants can play so that eating out doesn't contribute to our weight-related problems rather than help resolve them. See Chapter 12.

The Way Things Are

HOW OFTEN DO MOST TEENS EAT WITH THEIR FAMILIES?

A survey we did in Project EAT turned up great diversity in family meal patterns, as the following table shows.

A third of the families ate family meals only two or fewer times a week. But nearly half ate at least five meals together. On average, adolescents reported eating meals with "all or most" of their family living in their homes 4.5 times in the past week. We didn't ask about which meals they shared, so this

FREQUENCY OF FAMILY MEALS IN PAST WEEK AMONG TEENAGERS

Never	14%
One to two times	19%
Three to four times	21%
Five to six times	19%
Seven times	9%
More than seven times	18%

The data from Neumark-Sztainer D, Hannan PJ, Story M, Croll J, Perry C. Family meal patterns: associations with sociodemographic characteristics and improved dietary intake among adolescents. *Journal of the American Dietetic Association*. 2003; **3**: 317–322.

could have been breakfast together four or five times a week; breakfast before school and work on Monday, Sunday brunch, Saturday lunch, and two weeknight dinners; or it could have been dinner together every weeknight.

In focus group discussions, the teenagers' conversations clearly confirmed the diversity in family meal patterns. In some households, family meals were part of the daily routine, whereas in others the only routine was the lack of family meals because "no one's ever home." For kids whose parents didn't live together, sometimes there were family meals at one parent's house and none at the others. Some families ate dinner around the kitchen table, others ate in the living room in front of the TV (but together), and still others retreated to their respective quarters to eat while pursuing whatever activity each individual was absorbed in.

As you might expect, we found that older teens ate fewer family meals than younger teens. We also found that girls had fewer family meals than boys; this may have been due to more girls skipping meals for weight control purposes (45%) than boys (18%),

But here's my favorite finding: *Frequency of family meals hardly varied whether the mother was employed or not!* In our study, 68% of the mothers worked full-time, 22% worked part-time, and 10% were not employed. The average number of family meals during the past week was 4.2 in homes where the mother worked full-time, 4.5 in homes where the mother worked part-time, and 4.9 in homes where the mother was not employed.

So, no need to give up your job *or* smother yourself in guilt for not gathering the clan for every meal. Most of us working mothers probably couldn't afford to give up our jobs—even if we wanted to. Being employed outside the home may make it more difficult to get dinner on the table, but it clearly isn't telling the whole story. What does?

WHAT GETS IN THE WAY OF FAMILY MEALS?

• **Busy schedules.** Teens who participated in our research studies mentioned busy or conflicting schedules of parents and teenagers more frequently than any other reason for not participating in family meals. Parents may still be at work during mealtimes, and teens are often away from home at sports, extracurricular school activities, work, and socializing. For some families this may mean dining in the car on the way to a soccer game, in other families this means everyone for himself searching in the freezer for something to pop in the microwave, while for better-organized families, this may mean cooking up a pot of soup or a pan of lasagna that everyone can eat from whenever they get home. These findings suggest a need for greater distribution of meal preparation responsibilities. They also suggest a need for rethinking family schedules and priorities; although some activities have to take priority over family meals, others can possibly be shifted around. Creativity is also important; family breakfasts or brunches may work better than family dinners.

- **A desire to be independent.** Another frequently mentioned reason for not participating in family meals was a desire for autonomy. Teens discussed wanting to be on their own or with friends. If they were out with friends, they didn't want to have to come home to eat. If this is the case in your house, solutions that might work here include negotiating a number of times that you do want your teen home for dinner, having certain nights where everyone is expected to be home, or opening up family dinners to your teens' friends (at least sometimes).

- **Dissatisfaction with family relations at meals.** Another reason for avoiding family meals was dissatisfaction with family relations around the table. Some teens objected to having to listen to their parents tell them what to eat. Others disliked having to answer all of their parents' questions at meals. Rather than no longer asking teens questions at meals, the solution may be to avoid the questions or topics that are likely to lead to conflict.

- **Just don't like the food.** A less frequently mentioned reason for not wanting to eat with one's family related to the taste or type of food served. Some teens just prefer fast foods.

Does any of this sound familiar? I bet it does. We all face the same obstacles. It's interesting, then, that no matter whom I talk to, when the topic of family meals comes up, everyone expresses feeling a bit guilty about not being able to pull it off all the time. Maybe that's because it's something our parents did, seemingly without effort. Even if not, though, I think almost everyone instinctively feels that losing the family meal tradition is robbing us of something valuable. And as much as they complained about family meals feeling like command performances, being grilled at dinner, or not liking the food, teens tended to agree.

WHAT TEENS LIKE ABOUT FAMILY MEALS

- **A little stability in often chaotic lives.** One girl said that eating dinner as a family was one of the only things about her eating that's always been constant and called it "another part of the day."

cantly more calcium, iron, folate, and other important vitamins and minerals; and have fewer ready-made dinners (such as frozen dinners, Spaghetti Os, and microwave meals).

- **Lower body mass index (BMI).** Studies suggest that teens who eat more frequently with their families have lower BMI values (weight for height) and are less likely to be overweight.

- **Less alcohol, tobacco, and marijuana use.** Family meals provide an opportunity for touching base with our teens on a regular basis. Maybe that accounts for the fact that our research team found that teens who eat more often with their families use less tobacco, alcohol, and marijuana. Among other findings, this one really stood out: *Nearly half of the girls who did not eat family meals reported smoking, in comparison to only 19% of the girls who had daily family meals.*

- **Higher grades in school.** Lower-than-average grades were reported by 57% of the girls and 63% of the boys who ate no meals with their families, a compared with 42% of girls and 48% of boys who ate seven or more family meals.

- **Lower rates of depression and fewer suicidal thoughts and actions.** A high level of depressive symptoms was reported by 49% of the girls who had no family meals and 32% of the boys, as compared with 31% of the girls and 17% of the boys who ate at least seven family meals. Suicide attempts were double among those who had no family meals—21% versus 9% for the girls and 10% versus 6% for the boys.

- **Fewer disordered eating behaviors.** In a study of college women, those who had eaten on a more regular basis with their families before going off to college were at lower risk for bulimia nervosa at college. Even in families with strained relationships, family meals appeared to have benefits. In Project EAT we found a similar association: nine percent of adolescent girls who ate meals with their families five or more times in the past week used extreme weight control behaviors, as compared with 18% of girls who ate with their families two or fewer times. *Disordered eating decreased sharply in teens reporting at least three to four family meals a week.*

This doesn't mean that all teenagers who eat infrequently with their families will engage in disordered eating behaviors. But the findings do tell us that family meals may have a protective effect against eating disorders, possibly because they provide opportunities for parents to model healthy eating patterns and provide healthier foods, and because if they're not at meals together, parents may not have the chance to notice a teen's budding eating disorder.

Ask your teenagers and other fa
members to describe family meal
your home. If they use words like
quent, pleasant, fun, relaxing, and to
and they talk fondly about special fa

ily rituals, keep doing what you're doing. If not, don't get down on yourse
but do think about where you could make some changes. What woul
need to happen to get your teen to describe family meals in your home in
a way you would like?

- **Traditional family foods.** When asked to name their favorite food
and whom they usually eat it with, surprisingly few teens said, "Pizza, with
friends." Rather, many said things like "fried chicken and collard greens with
my family," "fish at family fish fries," "tamales at my great-grandma's house,"
"roast that I eat with my family," "steak when my family goes out on Sundays," and "enchiladas that my mom makes all spicy."

- **Holidays and other family rituals.** The teens also talked very positively about family meals associated with holidays, birthdays, family gatherings,
or other special events. Many kids named foods served at these celebrations as
their favorite foods. Teens also liked family rituals such as gatherings on Sundays, restaurant meals after church with the family, and making a special family
meal one day a week. So, even if you can't all eat together most of the time,
there are a host of possibilities for creating new rituals around family meals.

What would fit in with your family
style and schedule? Sunday brunch
after working out, going to church,
or just sleeping in? Summer barbe-

cues? Spaghetti on Tuesdays, with friends invited? Friday night dinner as
the week comes to an end? Sunday evenings before the week begins?

The Way Things *Could* Be

Let's imagine the possibilities: Exactly what might our teenagers get out of it
if we could provide more family meals?

- **Better eating habits.** Teenagers who eat more meals with their families eat more fruits, vegetables, and grains; drink less soda pop; take in signifi-

FAMILY MEALS: THE MIRACLE CURE FOR ALL TEENAGE WOES?

If you're thinking that all of this sounds too good to be true and must be due to something else going on in families, so were we. But we did a special statistical analysis and found that *family meals make a difference above and beyond overall family connectedness.* Thus, even if family relations in your home are less than ideal, family meals may help, perhaps through increased monitoring of your teen's whereabouts, more knowledge about your teen's behaviors and mood states, and more family conversations. If family members at your home tend to have pretty good relationships, eating together more often may also have a positive impact on your teen, via similar processes of monitoring and staying in touch.

I don't want to overstate the case here. Based our findings, we can say that family meals are strongly associated with a range of measures of adolescent well-being. But we don't know what comes first—the lack of family meals or the problematic adolescent behaviors. We think the influence goes mainly from family meals to adolescent behaviors, but it may work in the other direction too: teens who are smoking pot, feeling depressed, or following a strict diet may just not come to the table. Stay tuned for findings from Project EAT–II, which is currently under way.

How You Can Reap the Benefits of Family Meals without Spending Your Life in the Kitchen

Close your eyes for a moment and picture your ideal family meal. What do you see? The first image I see is a family scene out of *Leave It to Beaver.* Ward, June, Wally, and the Beav are sitting around a home-cooked meal, which began at 6:30 sharp, discussing the day's events. The food is tasty and nutritious, the kids are respectful, the conversation is interesting, and the atmosphere is relaxed and free of conflict.

Okay, now forget about that image.

There are steps you can take to reap the benefits of family meals without stepping through the looking glass à la the 1998 movie *Pleasantville.*

I. START WITH SMALL CHANGES IN THE FREQUENCY OF FAMILY MEALS

You'll get overwhelmed if you try to make huge changes in your family's meal routines. Start small. Just try to have one more family meal together than you usually do. And make it an easy one. Can it be an informal breakfast or brunch on Saturday or Sunday? Or a midweek "pasta night"—on whatever day your family has the fewest scheduled activities?

In the two weeks following the completion of our study of family meals and disordered eating, my family was just raving about the fancy cooking I was doing. But last night when I was trying to make some progress on this chapter, I ordered in pizza for my family. *C'est la vie.*

In my home we still don't all meet for family dinners as often as I'd like, for the same reasons cited by the teens in our focus groups. But we nearly always eat a traditional meal together on Friday nights as we welcome in the Jewish Sabbath. When a television reporter came to my office to interview me about my research on family meals in the homes of teenagers, I invited him to come film a Friday night dinner at our home. We were having a lively meal with lots of tasty and traditional foods. He passed around a microphone to each of my four children and asked them what they thought about family meals, in particular about our ritual of eating together on Friday evenings. Their positive comments took me somewhat by surprise. Tal said his parents' expectations for him to be home for dinner make him feel important and cared about. Lior, who goes to a nearby university, talked about how there were times during high school when he didn't want to come home for meals, but now he could see how important family meals are. He votes with his feet; even though he doesn't live at home, he comes around most Friday nights for dinner.

Such rituals are important and often pay disproportionate returns to the whole family. But my goal, based on all the research, mine and that of other scientists, is this:

Aim for at least three to four family meals a week. That's not an arbitrary number, but based on the finding that disordered eating decreased sharply in teens reporting at least three to four family meals a week. And it's a lot less daunting than trying to get the whole family together every single day.

---

what you can do
SHARE THE WORK

Are you a working parent? Creativity and flexibility may be needed to make family meals happen in your home. How about assigning the kids the task of cooking once a week? Let them pick the menu—*as long as it's home cooked, within reason.* This may mean no take-outs, delivery pizza, or fast food. But it could include jarred pasta sauce and bagged salad mixtures.

Our research has motivated me to change things in our family to make family meals more frequent, nutritious, pleasant, and structured. As much as possible, we try to avoid working or engaging in other activities in the evening so that we eat a minimum of three to four meals together a week. I ask my kids for ideas about what they would like to eat at dinner. And, for the most part, we have been successful in postponing topics likely to lead to conflict to after the meal.

Why are these factors important? Because studies have shown that the quality of the time spent together at family meals and the structured routine also contribute to the benefits that teenagers get from them.

2. TRY TO MAKE FAMILY MEALTIMES QUALITY TIME

To assess the atmosphere at family meals, we asked teenagers to indicate how strongly they agreed with the statements in the following table. Try answering the questions for your family. Circle the numbers that best describe the atmosphere at family meals and add them up. Scores can range from 4 (negative atmosphere) to 16 (positive atmosphere); higher scores suggest a more enjoyable atmosphere.

HOW ENJOYABLE ARE FAMILY MEALS IN YOUR HOME?

	Strongly disagree	Somewhat disagree	Somewhat agree	Strongly agree
1. I enjoy eating meals with my family.	1	2	3	4
2. In my family, mealtime is a time for talking with other family members.	1	2	3	4
3. In my family, dinnertime is about more than just getting food; we all talk with each other.	1	2	3	4
4. In my family, eating brings people together in an enjoyable way.	1	2	3	4

From *"I'm, Like, SO Fat!"* by Dianne Neumark-Sztainer. Copyright 2005 by Dianne Neumark-Sztainer.

Not surprisingly, teens who reported a positive atmosphere at family meals in their homes were less likely to engage in disordered eating behaviors.

For example, 18% of girls who reported a very negative atmosphere at meals (scores close to 4) engaged in uncontrolled binge eating, as compared with 8% of girls who reported a very positive atmosphere at family meals (scores close to 16).

Quality, not just quantity, counts. But if mealtime at your home is anything but a scene out of *Pleasantville,* don't despair. Aim for small steps toward high-quality family meals, just as you do with frequency.

what you can do
AVOID HOT-BUTTON TOPICS AND CRITICISM AT THE TABLE

During your few meals together, avoid making comments likely to make your teen feel bad or get mad, such as "Haven't you had enough?" or "How is your diet going?" or "Your room is a mess" or "We need to talk about your grades!" If your teen is eating too much or too little at dinner, don't get pulled into a heated discussion at the table; rather, bring up your concern later. And if your teen (or anyone) starts an argument at dinner, you can choose not to go there.

3. GIVE YOUR FAMILY ROUTINE SOME STRUCTURE

In Project EAT we asked teens how strongly they agreed with the statements shown in the table on the facing page. Again, try this out for your own family. Circle the numbers that best describe family meals at your home and add them up. The possible range for scores is 5 (low structure at family meals) to 20 (high structure at family meals). The higher the number, the more structured family meals are in your own home.

Our findings suggested that teens who came from homes with more structured meals were less likely to engage in disordered eating, suggesting that parents should have certain rules, such as requiring that children eat at the table, use appropriate table manners, and try new foods being served. Children should not be taking dinner into their bedrooms to eat alone with the television, as some teens in our study were doing.

But let's apply common sense here: Sitting around the table and using good manners makes sense, but I would not suggest making children eat foods they don't like or ever pushing kids to eat once they are full. I've stressed the principle of moderation throughout this book, and just as it wouldn't make sense to have no rules about family meals, going overboard with rules can be harmful as well.

HOW STRUCTURED ARE FAMILY MEALS IN YOUR HOME?

	Strongly disagree	Somewhat disagree	Somewhat agree	Strongly agree
1. In my family, there are rules at mealtimes that we are expected to follow.	1	2	3	4
2. Manners are important at our dinner table.	1	2	3	4
3. In my family, a child should eat all the foods served even if he or she doesn't like them.	1	2	3	4
4. In my family, we don't have to eat meals at the kitchen/dining room table.	4	3	2	1
5. In my family, it is okay for a child to make something else to eat if he or she doesn't like the food being served.	4	3	2	1

From *"I'm, Like, SO Fat!"* by Dianne Neumark-Sztainer. Copyright 2005 by Dianne Neumark-Sztainer.

what you can do
TWEAK THE ENVIRONMENT TO MAKE MEALS A LITTLE MORE STRUCTURED

Microwave ovens, island kitchens (instead of sit-around tables), competing activities, favorite television programs, and ringing phones can all get in the way of a family meal shared around the dining table. Can you think of one way to make meals a bit more structured in your home? A good place to start is by making some food that you know your kids like, telling them you're eating at 5:30 (or whenever), and cleaning off the kitchen table and setting it with plates, cups, and silverware, so that they realize you'll be sitting together tonight. How about turning down the volume on the phone closest to the table and letting your voice mail answer calls during dinner? Or making sure there's no TV within viewing distance of the table? If your kitchen has an island, is it big enough to put stools with backs on them around the island so you can have a pleasant meal there? Do you have a sheltered patio or deck where you can have your family meals during warm weather? How about a dining room table for distinguishing special family meals from the regular ones? Do you have some candles to light for a special atmosphere?

4. THINK ABOUT WHAT WOULD WORK FOR *YOUR* FAMILY

As a family, you need to decide:

1. What is important to you in terms of eating patterns and family meals?
2. What do you like about family meals in your home?
3. What would you like to change?
4. What are going to be your first steps?

Take a moment to write down what you like about family meals in your home and what you'd like to change. I've done it for my family; feel free to steal any similarities.

WHAT KINDS OF THINGS DO YOU LIKE ABOUT FAMILY MEALS IN YOUR HOME? WHAT WOULD YOU LIKE TO CHANGE?

What do you like?	What would you like to change?	What are some ideas for making change happen?

From *"I'm, Like, SO Fat!"* by Dianne Neumark-Sztainer. Copyright 2005 by Dianne Neumark-Sztainer.

THINGS I LIKE ABOUT FAMILY MEALS AT MY HOME AND THINGS I WOULD LIKE TO CHANGE

Things I like	Things I would like to change	Ideas for making change happen
We eat a good dinner together nearly every Friday night and have rituals associated with the Jewish Sabbath.	Before going shopping, we think about what we want to make for Friday night dinner, but don't always do this for the rest of the week.	We can talk about a few dinner ideas before going grocery shopping to be better prepared.
Our dinner discussions are often very vibrant.	Sometimes the discussions are too vibrant and turn into arguments.	When things get heated up, I need to say clearly, "Let's talk about this after dinner."
Everyone knows they need to sit at the table to eat if they are home and awake.	We do not eat dinner together as frequently as I would like since we have a lot going on.	In the morning, I need to remind my kids that we want to eat dinner together tonight, that I am making chicken and rice (their favorite), and that we'll be eating at 7:30.
We usually have salad and rarely have fried foods.	Different family members have different food likes and dislikes, and in appealing to the lowest common denominator, things can get boring.	I am going to suggest that we make one "new thing" (or an old thing with a new recipe) once a week and get ideas from other family members on foods they would like to try.
My family is appreciative of the cook (usually my husband or me).	I would like my kids to be more involved in food preparation.	I am going to suggest that we do one night of "kid cooks in the kitchen" or see if anyone has another suggestion.

Change is difficult, and it's better to succeed with small changes one at a time than to fail at larger changes. Take a look at your list and decide on one thing you like about family meals in your home that you would like to continue and strengthen. Now choose one thing you dislike that you would like to change. If you think it will be helpful, discuss this change with your family. There are many good ideas, some of which you've already read about in this chapter:

1. Aim to eat one more family meal a week.
2. Shoot for at least three to four family meals a week.
3. Promote a positive atmosphere by avoiding discussions of topics likely to lead to arguments. If conflicts arise, try not to get caught up in them and clearly state that the "hot" topic should be discussed after the meal is completed.
4. Avoid weight-related comments, and discuss concerns about how much or how little others are eating at another time.
5. Insist that your teenagers come to the table for family meals; don't allow them to eat in their rooms or in front of the TV by themselves.
6. Avoid being a short-order cook. Try to have one food item that everyone likes, but accept the fact that not everyone is going to like everything all the time.
7. Before signing up your child for another extracurricular activity, think about the impact it will have on family meals in your home.
8. When things are just too hectic, eating out in a restaurant can provide a respite. No cooking is necessary, and your kids will have to sit at the table. In the next chapter we explore how to avoid some of the nutritional pitfalls of eating out.

what you can do
ADVOCATE FOR CHANGE BEYOND YOUR FRONT DOOR

The frequency and quality of family meals is not determined by familial factors only. After-school sports influence teens, and heavy work demands and work schedules may keep parents away from home over the dinner hour. Community and societal factors draw teens away from families at mealtimes by making it easy to grab something to eat on the run and deemphasizing the importance of family meals (see Chapter 2).

Is there anything you can do to advocate for changes in social norms regarding family meals? At a PTA meeting, can you suggest that sports events be scheduled outside dinnertime? How about suggesting that the school newspaper run an editorial on the subject? In organizing an end-of-the season sports party, can you suggest that all family members be invited if it includes a meal (and does so at a reasonable cost)? At work, can you suggest that going out for a drink with co-workers be scheduled for four o'clock, because you like to be home to have dinner with your family? One of my colleagues used our research findings as a basis for planning PTA and Girl Scout parent meetings after the dinner hour (which tends to be early in Minnesota). It can be done!

12

Eating Out—When Cooking Just Isn't Going to Happen

*H*ow ironic. How timely. Just as I'm beginning to think about how to write this chapter, I'm stuck in a roadside McDonald's. I'm on vacation in Israel with my family, and we've rented a car to drive down south to Eilat. Our car got not one but two flat tires en route. Since it's Saturday, most restaurants are closed; the only place open here in this roadside center is McDonald's. Good thing for them, because the place is full of families with young children and teenagers. They're eating Happy Meals, meal deals in different sizes, and all the rest. There are a few differences in menu items: They don't serve cheeseburgers, and I was able to get a decent cup of cappuccino. Otherwise, the menu is the standard American one.

When I look around, I think it's great that these families can get out for an easy meal and spend time talking together in an informal atmosphere. The kids are happy—and therefore so are their parents. This is one of the great things about eating out: Everyone can relax. I sure am glad this McDonald's is open, because we're stuck here for a few hours and no one cares that my teens are sitting at the next table playing cards after having some fries and drinks. Yet, I can't help wondering what all the other patrons would be doing and eating if McDonald's didn't exist in Israel. When I lived here about 10 years ago, it didn't. Would families be eating freshly cooked meals with a variety of salads at home? Would the quality of family interactions be different? Would the children be getting different messages about "mealtimes"? Would the meal include less fat and more fiber?

I'm going to let you in on a writer's secret. This chapter was not included in my original book outline. But when my editors reviewed an initial draft of the preceding chapter on family meals . . . well, let's just say that I could feel the tension rising. Perhaps you felt the same way when you read that chapter. As busy working women and mothers of teenagers, they had found that one solution for getting their families together was to go out to eat. They talked about how being out really allowed them to relax and talk with their teens. They put a further positive spin on something that I've also found works for my family . . . and for me when I'm just not in the mood for cooking and cleaning up. Sure, it would be great to have home-cooked family meals at least once a day, but that's not a reality for many of today's families.

Eating out can be a wonderful option for families. It can be a way to get your family together. No one needs to cook. People need to behave. And everyone usually sits and talks for more than 10 minutes. But there are drawbacks, as I'm sure you know: large portion sizes, hidden fat and calories, and free refills on soft drinks.

Fortunately they can be avoided so that you can get all the benefits of eating out without throwing in the towel on healthy eating practices.

WHY EAT OUT?

- **Eating out can be a way to increase the frequency of family meals** when you're too busy to even think about frying an egg, unable to come up with an idea of what to make for dinner, fed up with not getting to sit down and talk with your kids because of ringing telephones and competing activities, and tired of being the chief cook and pot scrubber. Get everyone in the car or tell your teens to meet you at a local restaurant at seven o'clock for a free dinner. You can sit with your family instead of serving them. You can avoid having family arguments, because others are looking. Everyone gets to choose what he or she wants to eat. And if you get everyone to turn off the cell phones, you might be able to get through a meal without outside interruptions.

- **Eating out provides an opportunity for you to connect with your teens.** Whether with your entire family or just your teen, meeting for a meal in a restaurant can provide a great setting for talking. Chapter 11 described the research data showing that teens who have more meals with their families eat healthier, smoke less, get better grades, and engage in fewer disordered

YES, WE ARE EATING OUT MORE OFTEN ...

What you might guess is true: Eating out is not just for special occasions anymore. One of the most noticeable changes in eating patterns of Americans has been the increased popularity of eating out or purchasing foods prepared outside the home. Data from the National Restaurant Association and the United States Department of Agriculture that:

- Between 1977 and 1995, the percentage of meals and snacks eaten at fast-food restaurants increased 200%, and other restaurant use increased 150%.
- In 1955, 25% of food dollars in the United States were spent in restaurants; this rose to 47% in 2004 and is predicted to rise to 53% by 2010.
- About half (46%) of all adults were restaurant patrons on a typical day during 1998.
- The average teenager visits a fast-food restaurant twice a week, and fast-food outlets provide about one-third of the away-from-home meals consumed by teens.

When people ate out once a week, it didn't really matter what they ate in restaurants. But it does make a difference when eating out is a more regular practice. Some professionals attribute the increased prevalence of obesity to the changes that have occurred in eating-out patterns because of the large portions (see Chapter 9) and the high fat content of many restaurant foods.

eating behaviors. At least part of this is probably due to the interactions that happen around the table. Sometimes this table can be a restaurant table instead of your kitchen table.

- **Eating out can become one of those family rituals that your kids cherish.** A routine of regular family meals at home bestows a wealth of benefits, but we all like a break from our normal routine. Maybe your Sunday brunch can be dim sum at your favorite Chinese restaurant. Or Friday dinner can be Italian night at the local trattoria that specializes in family-style dining and draws big, cheerful groups sharing platters of food. It doesn't have to be weekly, either. Maybe you can make a custom of celebrating with an informal dinner out whenever you have something to celebrate: a great report card, a sports victory, a birthday, or your teen getting his driver's license (kind of a mixed celebration).

- **A change of scene is a good place to introduce a variety of foods.** Variety is not just the spice of life but the backbone of good nutrition. Going out can broaden the range of foods your family eats. Kids who balk at vegetables at home might try them if they're in a Greek soup, on top of Italian pizza, or in a Chinese stir-fry. Reluctant legume eaters may be willing to eat beans in a burrito at a Mexican restaurant, lentils with some great spices at an Indian restaurant, or falafel with hummus at an Israeli restaurant. Encourage them to try something different, but don't force they them to eat something they don't like.

what you can do
HELP YOUR KIDS RELISH WHAT THEY EAT BY MAKING FOOD AN ADVENTURE

In my opinion, all too often when we talk about food, we talk about the "shoulds" and "shouldn'ts" of food choices. Food should be relished as we eat it and appreciated as an integral part of every culture. Eating out in different ethnic restaurants can be a path for exploring the world and broadening our children's understanding of different cultures. Share with them the excitement of trying something brand new.

- **Eating out demonstrates the importance of flexibility in eating habits.** When you go to a restaurant, whether it's a fast-food operation, a four-star temple of haute cuisine, or something in between, the menu will limit your choices and make it pretty impossible to dictate precisely what will pass your lips. This may mean having your steak cooked in a way you're not used to—or having red meat for the second time this week even though you "should" have fish or chicken. Demonstrating flexibility and expecting your teens to go with the flow, too, reinforces the idea that rigidity and restrictions should not govern our eating.
- **Eating out provides you with an opportunity to observe your teen's eating patterns.** If worries about your teen's eating habits are lurking in the back of your mind, being in a restaurant can give you a chance to observe informally. Is your teen unduly picky about her order, ordering no dressing on her salad or asking exactly how much oil is used in cooking the fish she wants? Does she eat her food slowly and with enjoyment, just push it around her plate, or wolf it down like it's her last meal? Is your teen sharing the appetizers ordered for the table or just watching others eat? Does she have some

bread before eating? Use a bit of butter—or much more than you've ever seen her use at home? What about dessert? Your observations will give you some information for a conversation *at a later time*.

- **Eating out can help your teen establish meal patterns.** Is your teen a grazer? Is your teen always nibbling and never really hungry for meals? I know that it helps if I can gently remind my kids that at seven o'clock we're going out for dinner. I hope that they will then think to themselves, "I should save some room so that I'll be able to enjoy my meal."

WHY EXERCISE A BIT OF CAUTION WHEN YOU DO GO OUT?

- **Food portions at today's restaurants tend to be huge, requiring an active effort to avoid overeating.** As discussed in Chapter 9, portion sizes have increased in all types of restaurants—including fast-food and family-style places.

- **You can't be sure what's in the food you're ordering, but you can be fairly sure that at many restaurants—fast-food and others—it includes a lot more fat and, possibly, sugar than you might cook with at home.** For example, the Center for Science in the Public Interest found that a standard eight-ounce serving of garlic bread that can be ordered in Italian restaurants has 820 calories and 40 grams of fat. An order of fettucine Alfredo (2.5 cups) has 1,500 calories and 97 grams of fat. At a typical Chinese restaurant, an order of General Tso's chicken has 1,600 calories and 59 grams of fat. Restaurant muffins have about 500 calories, mainly because they tend to be so big and have a fair amount of fat in them. Cinnabons, whose delicious smell permeates shopping malls, contain a whopping 670 calories each.

---

what you can do
MAKE MODERATION THE RULE

Would I advise you never to order garlic bread at an Italian restaurant? Of course not. The message of this book is *moderation*—this is what we want to achieve in the prevention of the broad spectrum of weight-related problems. Order the garlic bread sometimes. Get one order and share with everyone at the table. And when you eat it, *be sure to enjoy it*. One of the problems is that people eat a lot and then feel guilty about it. This totally defeats the purpose of having a good dinner. Furthermore, this type of thinking can feed into behaviors such as bingeing followed by purging or binge-diet-binge cycling.

<table>
<tr><td>

what you can do
KNOW WHAT
THE HEALTHIER CHOICES
ARE IN VARIOUS CUISINES

</td><td>

Sometimes (not always; see the "Make Moderation the Rule" box on p. 206) opt for these menu items instead of the garlic bread, fettuccine Alfredo, General Tso's chicken, or mega-muffin:

</td></tr>
</table>

➜ Have plain Italian bread or breadsticks—about one-fifth the fat of garlic bread.

➜ Choose spaghetti with marinara sauce—about half the calories and less than a fifth of the fat of the Alfredo.

➜ In place of General Tso's chicken, try stir-fried vegetables—750 calories and 19 grams of fat.

➜ Instead of the Godzilla-sized muffin, choose a smaller version. Better yet, eat a bagel, toast, or an English muffin.

For more hits on eating out healthfully, check out the Center for Science in the Public Interest's website on restaurants: *www.cspinet.org/restaurant/index.html*. Take its quiz "Rate Your Restaurant Diet." It's fun and informative.

SHOULD FAST FOOD BE BANNED?

Okay, that was a trick question. By now you know that I don't think *any* food should be completely banned from one's diet. Position fast foods as "sometimes" foods when you talk to your kids about them to avoid extreme views—most fast foods are okay to eat sometimes. But I do think teenagers should be persuaded to make fast food the exception instead of the rule. Here's how Project EAT found that teens who had eaten fast food at least three times in one week compared to those who hadn't eaten any:

• Girls ate 100% more cheeseburgers, and boys 73% more.
• Girls ate 60% more french fries, and boys 53% more.
• Girls drank 45% more soft drinks, and boys 42% more.
• Both consumed one-fourth to one-third less fruit, vegetables, and milk.

Who are these kids? Could be yours—one-fourth of the teens we surveyed had eaten fast food at least three times in the past week, one-half one or two times, and one-fourth not at all.

Considering these food items, it should be no surprise that teens who ate more foods from fast-food restaurants had higher caloric intakes, and that more of their calories came from fat, than teens who ate fewer fast foods. Another

Eating Out

study confirmed that not eating fast food makes a difference: Dr. Bowman and colleagues found that children and teens consumed 126 fewer calories a day, and had better dietary intakes, on days when they did not eat in fast-food restaurants.

what you can do PROVIDE FAST-FOOD TIPS FOR YOUR TEENS	Obviously you can't control what your teens eats when he is on his own in a fast-food restaurant (or, for that matter, when you are with him). Your best

bet is to model healthy choices when you are with him. But here are some tips that you may find useful:

→ Remind your teen that fast food is *not* an essential food group and does not need to be part of a daily diet.

→ If your teen's school has an open-campus policy during lunchtime, I strongly advise against providing money for your teen to visit the local McDonald's on a regular basis.

→ Help your teen realize that the more-for-your money route is not always the best value in terms of health.

→ Free refills on soft drinks are a good financial deal ... but their high caloric content and total lack of nutrients don't make them a good deal for your teen's weight and overall health. Suggest that your teen go easy on refills—or better yet, get juice or milk.

→ There are a lot of teen-friendly fast-food places that offer pasta, salads, vegetables to add to sandwiches, vegetarian options, and low-fat deli meats. Encourage your teen to choose places that offer a variety of foods and when at those places to at least eat something green!

How to Make Eating Out Healthy and Enjoyable

Take a few moments to think about your own family's eating-out practices. Is there anything you'd like to change? Choose one or two of the ideas from the list below (or from what you've read in this chapter so far) to adopt, or come up with one or two ideas of your own. Think about how you choose a restaurant, order food, eat, talk about eating, and use the time when eating out to connect with family members. Is there room for improvement? If your family eats out only on special occasions, enjoy, splurge, and don't give it a second thought. These ideas are for families who eat out more frequently.

CHOOSING THE RESTAURANT

- Put different family members in charge of choosing the restaurant at different times, but emphasize trying a variety of ethnic cuisines.
- Think twice about choosing to go to a buffet. These can be great for teens with large appetites and for families on the run. But they can encourage excessive eating and may not allow time for sitting and chatting.
- Choose restaurants that offer healthy options. Most, but not all, do. Chinese food can be one great way to go—if you go heavy on the steamed rice, order foods with descriptions with include *stir-fried*, and limit your intake of fried breaded foods. But, as mentioned earlier, there are still better and worse choices within this cuisine, like any other.
- Want fast food? Fortunately, there's a new category of not-quite-as-fast-food restaurants that provide a variety of food choices and a place to sit comfortably and talk for at least 15 minutes. Restaurants such as Noodles & Company, Big Bowl, Panera Bread, and Chipotle seem to be springing up everywhere and are attractive to both teens and their families.

ORDERING ONCE YOU'RE THERE

- Feel free to ask the server for "special" orders, but don't go overboard. Demonstrating flexibility in eating patterns is important.
- It's good to know a *bit* about the nutrient and caloric content of foods served in restaurants. To educate your kids, say something like "I just read that fettuccine Alfredo has five times as much fat as spaghetti with marinara sauce. Since I like them both, I think I'll go with the marinara." Again, don't go overboard here or talk about it too much.
- Encourage your children to try different foods. If they aren't sure they'll like something, offer to share with them.
- Don't comment on a food that your teen orders unless asked; even a sensitive remark is bound to result in hurt feelings or a miserable meal.
- When ordering, look for words on the menu such as *baked, broiled, stir-fried, steamed,* and *grilled*. Go easy on foods that are described as *fried, buttery, crispy, creamy,* or *breaded*.
- To cut down on portion sizes, dinner costs, and food waste, consider sharing. Split an entrée with your teen or order a few entrées for the table and eat "Chinese style."

- Model healthy eating patterns when eating out. This is definitely a time when your children will pay attention to what you're eating. Eat a diversity of foods (not just salad or just burgers); select whole grains, fruits, vegetables, and dairy foods whenever possible; limit (but don't eliminate) fats and sugars; eat appropriate portion sizes; and enjoy what you eat.
- If you want an appetizer, go with soup, salad, or plain bread or share the garlic bread, fried mozzarella sticks, or calamari.
- Does your plate look like the food guide pyramid? Think about your meal and go heavy on whole grains, fruits, and vegetables.
- On sandwiches or burgers, use mustard or ketchup instead of mayonnaise or butter. This is an easy change that you won't even notice.
- Be aware of how large the portions are in some restaurants and eat according to your needs—not the restaurant's needs to attract customers by offering "good deals."
- If you can't share a large portion, take home a doggie bag.
- Don't try to get your money's worth with as many refills on soda pop as are possible.
- Share desserts. A bit of a dessert can finish the meal nicely and demonstrate that it's possible to enjoy foods from the tip of the pyramid in moderation.
- Eat until you're full or almost full. Pay attention to internal signs of hunger. We don't always have to leave a restaurant feeling totally stuffed.
- Eat slowly and savor the tastes.

YOU'RE ALSO THERE TO TALK

- If you do overeat, try to avoid saying things like "Why did I eat so much?" or "I feel sick from eating so much" or "I feel so bloated." If you feel as though you ate too much, make a note of it for next time but don't talk about it afterward. The idea is to demonstrate positive attitudes toward eating—and eating without guilt.
- Be particularly careful not to make comments likely to make your teens feel bad about their weight or food choices if you want them to join you again.

- Talk about how good the food is. Tell food stories associated with family traditions or travel. Demonstrate enjoyment of eating.
- Although you don't want to nag your teens about their eating patterns when eating out, this can be a "teaching moment" about nutrition. The best way is through modeling, but you can also share tidbits of knowledge that you've accumulated from this book or other sources. Try limiting them to one or two tidbits per meal.
- Avoid topics likely to lead to conflict between family members. You know what they are for your family.
- Use eating out as a time to connect with your teens. Ask specific questions to find out what's going on in their lives, and tell them what's going on in yours. *The main reason for eating out is to have time to connect.*

AND MOST IMPORTANT

Above all—relax and enjoy the food and the company!

what you can do
BE A SMARTER EATER-OUTER

Going Italian?
- → Take a peek at the other tables before ordering to get a sense of portion size.
- → Salad and minestrone soup are great starters.
- → In general, a red pasta sauce is a better choice than a white one.

Going Chinese? Thai? Vietnamese?
- → Clear soups are great starters.
- → These are great places to eat delicious vegetables.
- → Stick with steamed rice instead of fried; see if brown rice is available.
- → Share food; you probably don't need an entrée for everyone.

Japanese for a change?
- → You can't go wrong with sushi and miso soup.
- → Udon soup can be a whole meal.

How about Middle Eastern?
- → Enjoy the salads as a starter or a main course.

→ Stuff a pita bread with hummus and lots of cucumbers and tomatoes.

→ Go with lean meats and fish.

Mexican tonight?

→ Go easy on the chips before you are served your main course.

→ Fajitas with lots of vegetables are a great choice.

→ Finally, a place where beans taste good.

Hitting the steakhouse?

→ Go with a smaller, leaner portion of meat.

→ A baked potato is your best side dish; ask for either sour cream or butter—on the side.

→ Try fish for a change and choose broiled or grilled instead of deep-fried.

In a rush or just feel like fast food?

→ Choose a place with healthier options—soups, salads, sandwiches.

→ Avoid the supersizes—go with the medium.

→ Leave off the mayo, but ask for extra veggies.

Sunday brunch?

→ Cereal, fruit, bagels, and eggs with whole wheat toast are good choices.

→ Get a side order of fruit with your eggs or pancakes instead of bacon, sausages, or a muffin.

→ Ask for the butter on the side if you get pancakes.

Just want coffee?

→ Go easy with the specialty coffees. This is one place where you might want to check out the calories (a 20-ounce skinny cappuccino has 141 calories and a 20-ounce caramel cooler has 538).

→ Go with the smaller sizes.

→ Consider having a bagel instead of a croissant to go with your coffee.

Going to the movies?

→ Go with the smaller sizes of popcorn and hold the butter.

→ Stay away from the large soda pop.

→ Just watch the movie ... you'll have enough money for dinner afterward.

| **what you can do**
SPEAK UP AND VOTE
WITH YOUR FEET | Taking advantage of the restaurant experience may require a little more thought than it used to, but the good news is that you can make it happen. |

Keep in mind, when you're about to throw up your hands in frustration over supersizing and high-fat, low-nutrient menu items, that the restaurant industry responds to consumer demands. In fact, as I write this, changes are happening and McDonald's is pledging to reduce its supersizes, probably as a result of consumer demands, potential lawsuits, movies (*Supersize Me: A Film of Epic Portions,* by Morgan Spurlock), and negative publicity. Let your voice be heard in regard to the types of foods you think should be served in the restaurants you visit. Use your feet and your consumer power by avoiding restaurants that do not provide healthier options because their profit margins are smaller. Talk these decisions over with your teens; they may also decide to be consumer-savvy. If eating out is to be a norm, let's try to make it a healthy norm.

13

Fluent in the F Words

*Talking with Teens about Food, Fat,
and Other Touchy Topics*

*T*hroughout this book I've stressed that you'll have the greatest influence on your children's weight-related issues without saying a word. The loudest messages you can send come from what you do and not what you say. But in the very real world of your home, a lot of talking goes on. And how you talk about food and eating, body image and weight, activity and health, has a significant impact on your teens' risks of developing a weight-related problem. How you respond verbally when you're concerned about your teens' attitudes or behaviors or when a weight-related problem does come up makes a big difference in the outcome.

In this chapter I'll show you how just a few words can transform a message from somewhat negative to very positive. I'll offer some *do's* and *don'ts* that can open your teens to what you have to say instead of slamming the door on communication, and I'll provide some suggestions for how to react productively when the typically touchy subjects and situations arise between you.

BE PROACTIVE: ESTABLISH A HEALTHY HOME BASE THROUGH POSITIVE COMMUNICATION

One of the clearest and most consistent findings in research studies is that teens who feel connected to their parents are happier, healthier, and more successful in school in general. Where weight-related issues are concerned, a large research study found that teens who reported high levels of family communication and family caring were at one-third the risk for engaging in extreme weight control behaviors such as vomiting or using diet pills, laxatives, or diuretics. And your kids *will* seek you out when they have questions. In another large study more than half (58%) of the teenage girls and close to half of the boys (42%) said they'd go to their mothers first for information about health-related issues. Interestingly, only 18% of the girls and 10% of the boys said they would turn first to their friends. Although older teens were more likely to turn to their friends than younger children, parents remained the main source of information on health care issues throughout the teenage years.

Does this mean you have carte blanche for using the *F* words—*food, fitness,* and *fat*? Of course not. But it does mean that you have the right and the responsibility to talk about these issues with your kids. The trick is finding ways to do so that will create a healthy home base, not an atmosphere of criticism and shame. Teens in our research studies showed us that supportive and informative discussions about sensitive topics like weight, calories, and food intake are useful, but making them feel bad about themselves and their food choices nullifies any positive effects. Consider these *do*'s and *don't*s:

- **Avoid saying anything that might inadvertently shame your teen.** Saying "Do you know how many calories are in that Reuben sandwich you ordered?" at a restaurant will probably do more harm than good. Instead, wait until another time to provide some information on calories and nutrient density of different foods: "I've been reading this book about healthy and less healthy restaurant choices. Would you be interested in looking at it? It has some good information about which foods tend to be high in nutrients, but not excessive in calories."

- **Avoid comments like "I think you've had enough to eat"** and instead put the control back in your teens' hands. "Are you still feeling hungry?" shows respect for their drive to become autonomous and reminds them to pay attention to their own internal signs of hunger and satiety.

- **Find out what's going on with your teenager and his or her social environment.** How many minutes do you spend each day in conversation with your teens? (This does not include saying things like "Clean up your room.") Do you know their thoughts about important topics, such as how they feel about their bodies, sexual relationships, substance use, weight stigmatization and other forms of discrimination, personal fears and self-doubts, and their hopes and dreams for the future? Maybe you don't know how to frame the questions or you're not sure you're ready to deal with the answers.

If not, you're not alone. A good strategy is just to ask without making assumptions about the answers. "What do you think about kids making themselves throw up after eating a lot? Do you know kids who have done this? Have you?" is more likely to lead to an honest response than "You would never make yourself throw up after eating too much, would you?" I'll bring up a bunch of common situations that make parents feel tongue-tied later in the chapter and offer some ideas for how to really talk about them. If you spend enough time communicating with your teens, the important issues will come up naturally, but only if a lot of your communication involves actively listening.

• **Stay tuned in to the individual characteristics and needs of your children.** I asked my son Tal how he thinks parents should communicate with their teens about important topics. He said parents really need to take into account their teen's personality, sensitivity to the topic, and likely reaction to the topic at hand. I couldn't have said it better myself. Thinking about this in advance will help you decide where and when to have a certain conversation, how far to push things, and how you'll stay calm if your teen seems likely to get upset.

• **Make it clear where you stand on issues surrounding weight, food, and body image.** Our role as parents is to serve as a buffer against broader social forces that may negatively impact our children, such as idealized thin images portrayed in the media and enticements to order larger portions than our energy requirements demand. Actively seek opportunities to counteract these messages. When you're watching television, say, for example, "I hate it when women portrayed as sexual objects are used to sell cars." When you hear your teens engaging in fat talk, ask, "What does that mean, to 'feel fat'? Why do you think people talk about weight so often?" Steer the conversation toward other ways to talk about how we feel and how we look.

• **Inject positive reinforcement into virtually every conversation.** They may seem tough, but teens often are struggling with their self-esteem and need a lot of reassurance. Find a quiet spot and write down as many nice things as you can about each of your children. Then make a point of inserting these into your conversations. Use words that have nothing to do with appearance—*creative, kind, generous, fun, good friend, caring, smart, organized, athletic, smart, hardworking, unique, special, musical, responsible, interesting, funny.* But also compliment their looks—*beautiful, handsome, stylish, classy, unique, attractive, shiny hair, bright eyes, good posture, great way of moving, strong, soft skin.* Stay away from words such as *thin, fabulous figure, great body.*

• **Be patient with their preoccupations. They're playing to an imaginary audience.** Kids with rapidly changing bodies tend to be preoccupied with themselves and naturally assume that everyone else is paying as much attention to their own bodies as they are. So when your daughter says, "Oh gross! I can't go out with this THING on my face," referring to a barely visible pimple, avoid criticizing her exaggeration. Just keep emphasizing the positive: "You always pick the right thing to wear." "You have a great sense of style." Remind her that others also have imperfections that people don't seem to notice or care about: "That girl that you said is the most popular in the class wears braces and has skin problems just like everyone else." And sometimes I find it is most helpful to avoid getting into it with your teen. After saying something short and sweet, just leave the room to do something else: "I think you look great. I'll be downstairs sorting mail if you need me."

• **Ask how weight-related issues are being addressed at school.** Find out what's going on in your son's or daughter's health class. Ask whether the debate team ever talks about issues like ethics in advertising. When your teenager has a chance to pick a current-events controversy for writing an essay for English or social studies, suggest one of the topics the two of you have discussed, such as regulations about food labeling, the causes of eating disorders, or how schools should handle weight-related teasing.

• **Change the way you casually talk about food, weight, and eating.** The following chart will help you spot problematic statements that many of us make and offers more constructive alternatives. What is one thing you can do differently to counteract negative social influences telling your teen to eat more, sit more, but weigh less? Choose a behavior that is important but not too hard to change. After you've succeeded, choose another one. I started with never making negative weight-related comments about myself in front of my teens. ("I look so fat in these pants.") I progressed to making positive comments. ("Not bad for a mother of four. . . . ")

NEW WAYS TO TALK ABOUT FOOD, FITNESS, AND FAT

Instead of . . .	Try this . . .
• Talking about dieting for quick weight loss . . . (For example, "I need to go on a diet to lose weight for that party next week.")	• Switch the focus to healthy weight management via the adoption of eating and activity behaviors that can be done on a long-term basis. (For example, "Did you know that dieting often makes teens gain weight, because they end up getting hungry and then overeating? What are some changes that you could make without going on a diet?") *(cont.)*

Instead of . . .	Try this . . .
• Talking about how many calories are in food . . . (For example, "Do you know how many calories are in a glass of milk?")	• Talk about nutrient density, that is, how many nutrients one gets for a certain amount of calories. (For example, "Milk has the same amount of calories as pop—but it's more filling and is full of protein, calcium, and a whole lot of other good stuff.")
• Talking about calories as if they are something "bad" . . . (For example, "There are so many calories in that!")	• Talk about calories as a measure of the energy we need to do the things we like to do (like breathe and talk and walk). Talk about balancing energy intake with expenditure. (For example, "All foods have calories . . . we just need to balance how much we take in with how active we are.")
• Talking about the latest low carb, or other, popular diets . . . (For example, I just read about this new diet. Hey, it can't hurt to try.)	• Talk about pyramid eating, why it makes sense, and brainstorm ideas for making it happen in your home. (For example, I'm staying away from those diets. I'm not interested in losing weight just to put it back on again, plus a few pounds. Instead, I'm looking for ways to eat more fruits and vegetables, substitute whole grains for refined grains, and cut down on the extras.")
• Talking about how you want to lose weight, or how your teen would look better at a lower weight . . . (For example, "If only I could lose five pounds . . . ")	• Demonstrate acceptance of different shapes and sizes—including your own! (For example, "I just love looking at the different shapes of the women in my dance class.") Put the focus on behaviors and let your weight (or your teen's weight) take care of itself.
• Talking about how much physical activity is needed to burn up the calories in a piece of cheesecake you are eating . . . (For example, "This is going to demand a whole morning at the gym!")	• Enjoy the slice of cheesecake you are eating and talk about how good it is. (For example, This cheesecake is absolutely delicious. I'm eating it slowly and I'm savoring every bite.)

(cont.)

Instead of . . .	Try this . . .
• Talking about how many calories you are burning up while working out with your teen . . .	• Talk about how being physically active is fun and makes you feel better—better mood, more energy, better posture, feel stronger and so forth. (For example, "After going for a walk in the evening, I have more energy for working on my book.")
• Talking about "feeling fat" or responding to your teen's fat feelings with suggestions for dietary changes . . .	• Find out what lies behind the "feeling fat." Remind yourself or your teen that "fat" is not a "feeling." What is the real feeling? Is it loneliness, sadness, low self-confidence? What might be some possible solutions?
• Falling into the "body comparison trap" and comparing your body with movie stars' . . . (For example, "I get so depressed reading fashion magazines.")	• Focus on the positives in your body and help your teen to do the same. (I'll say things like "I like the way I look in this outfit. It's a good style for me," or "You have a beautiful way of carrying yourself. Everyone always comments on your poise.")
• Making comments about how much people weigh . . . (For example, "She would be so attractive if she lost a bit of weight.)	• Promote the acceptance of different body sizes.") Talk with your teen about the similarities between weightism and other "isms" such as racism. (For example, "Do you think weightism goes on more than racism? What do you think can be done to prevent it?")
• Accepting images portrayed in the media as ideal . . . (For example, "My life would be so different if only I looked like her.")	• Question whether the images are real (or computerized to perfection), realistic for most people, healthy, or even attractive. (For example, "Can you believe that they expect us to think that we would look like that if we wore that makeup?")
• Suggesting that your teen go on a diet after being the victim of weight teasing . . .	• Make sure that your teen knows that you are there for him, love him, and that weight teasing is 100% unacceptable. In a completely separate conversation, you can talk about the adoption of healthier eating and physical activity behaviors—but not now! *(cont.)*

Instead of . . .	Try this . . .
• Making comments on how much your teen is eating . . . (For example, "Are you sure you want more? Don't you think you have had enough?")	• Don't say anything. At another time talk about how it is important to pay attention to whether or not one is hungry in deciding how much to eat. Observe your teen and ask your teen questions to see what might be lying behind the overeating: How are things going at school? With your friends? What do you worry about most?
• Commenting on how much, or what, your teen has ordered in a restaurant . . .	• Don't say anything. Next time, preempt overeating in restaurants by suggesting sharing an entrée. At another time, talk about how portion sizes have grown over the years and how important it is to pay attention to one's internal signs of hunger and not eat according to what the restaurant owner thinks is a suitable portion size.
• Making comments about how "bloated" you feel after a big meal . . . (For example, "I ate way too much. I feel sick.")	• Talk about how good the food was and how you enjoyed it. (For example, "Now that was a good meal!") Go heavy on the salad at your next meal or just eat a bit less.
• Commenting on your teen's latest binge . . . (For example, "This has got to stop. It's just going to make things worse for you.")	• Talk about, and demonstrate, healthier ways of dealing with stress, loneliness, and other painful emotions. (For example, "I have had the worst day! I'm going out for a walk and, I hope, will come back in a better mood.")
• Talking about food restrictions (For example, "I'm cutting fat out of my diet.") . . .	• Talk more about eating more fruits, vegetables, and whole grains. (For example, "I would like to see us all eating more fruits and vegetables. What should I buy at the store?")
• Eating and exercising for weight changes . . .	• Talk about eating for health . . . building stronger bones and muscles. Focus on the positive. (For example, "I'll have milk. My bones are thirsty.")
• Talking about what one "should" and "should not" be eating . . .	• Talk about "normal" eating, whereby one generally eats according to the pyramid with moderation, variety, and balance. But there are days when we eat too much and days when we eat too little and days when we eat a lot of chocolate. That's okay.

How can you communicate better with your teen about food, fat, and other touchy topics? Answer the questions in the following worksheet.

COMMUNICATING WITH YOUR TEEN: THINKING AHEAD ABOUT YOUR CHILDREN AND THEIR SURROUNDINGS

What has worked well in communicating with your teen in the past? (Place? time? style?)

_____

_____

What hasn't worked well that you would like to avoid?

_____

_____

What kinds of reactions might you expect from your teen when you bring up a sensitive topic? (For example, anger, denial.)

_____

_____

How will you respond to some possible reactions from your child? (For example, keep the discussion short, stop the conversation before things go too far, stay calm, stay on track, leave the door open for further conversation.)

_____

_____

What are some positive influences on your teen that you would like to reinforce? (For example, peer group involvement in sports or volunteer activities, peer norms that accept diversity, peer avoidance of unhealthy dieting behaviors.)

_____

_____

What will you say to reinforce these influences? (For example, "I think it's great that you ... ")

_____

_____

(cont.)

Food, Fat, and Other Touchy Topics

What are some negative influences on your teen that you would like to filter out? (For example, peer fat talk, magazine articles and television programs that place too much emphasis on appearance.)

_____

_____

What will you say to counteract these influences? (For example, give ideas for dealing with fat talk, talk about alternatives to dieting, comment on positive traits, not related to appearance, of various people.)

_____

_____

Know What to Say When Problems Arise

If you plan and communicate with the intention of fostering positive attitudes and feelings about weight and food in your teenagers, you may minimize the number of weight-related problems that arise. But some problems are inevitable, and it's a good idea to know how to respond when they do. Start with this foundation:

• **Plan ahead if you need to raise a touchy topic.** Some subjects are difficult to raise. Prepare yourself by thinking things through. Bounce some ideas off a friend who also has a teen, or even practice on a friend or your spouse. Use other resources such as books, health care providers, and school counselors.

• **If you're initiating the conversation, decide on its purpose up front.** If you're bringing up a touchy subject, is the purpose of the conversation to let your daughter know you're available to talk? to show your concern? to ask if she'd like to see a dietitian?

• **Find the right time to talk.** Instead of saying something right away when you notice a problem, wait until you're calm and relaxed. If you smell vomit in the bathroom, don't go exploding into your teen's room and ask what's going on. If you come home from work and find your teen sprawled out in front of the television with a bag of chips and a bottle of soda on the

carpet, first go upstairs, take a shower, change your clothes, and have a cup of tea. Think about what you want to say. Make sure it's also a good time for your teen to talk. Don't get into discussions on touchy topics when either of you is stressed or rushed. And when you do talk, you're better off not trying to fit everything into one conversation.

- **Leave the door open for further communication.** If you see any sign that the conversation isn't constructive, say something like "I'd like to talk about this some more tomorrow," "I may have some more questions that I'd like to ask," "I need to think about things a bit more; let's talk in a few days," or "It's getting late; let's go out for dinner tomorrow, just the two of us, and we can continue talking."

- **Listen to what your teen is saying and offer support before advice.** When children have grown into their teenage years, your role is no longer to fix everything for them. They probably already know the answer to their concerns and just need to talk then out to bring them to the surface. Listen with your whole body and give your teen your full attention. *Put more effort into understanding than into being understood.* Express your support. Ask your child for ideas about possible solutions and save your advice for a different conversation, or at least for much later in this one.

- **Don't take things personally—no matter what your teen says to you.** At least try not to. Keep the conversation focused on your child and meeting your child's needs. This can be tough. Believe me—I know.

- **If at all possible, wait for your teen to bring up the topic.** This is particularly important if your concern is excess weight. In that case your teen is likely to bring it up in one form or another. When he does, brainstorm some solutions. Encourage him to aim for gradual changes, and to concentrate on behavior and let his weight settle at what is healthiest. Ask how you can be of most help. *An important caveat:* Don't wait for your teen to broach the subject if you notice the warning signs of an eating disorder (see Chapter 15).

These are the guidelines that I've found lay a good foundation for any conversation with a teen about weight-related subjects. But do you know what you'll say once you're on the hot seat and your teen says, "I'm so fat" or "I hate my body" or "I'm going on a diet tomorrow"? The rest of this chapter offers some ideas that you can think about. Do any of these responses fit the needs of your family? What can you adapt? What would you do differently?

Tessa talks a lot about not being able to control her eating and feeling too fat. She really gets down on herself and seems to work herself into a slump. What can I say to help her?

Be glad your daughter has invited you in, and make yourself available to hear what's going on. Find out if the issue is really about food or weight or if there is an underlying concern: "How are things going in your life? How have you been feeling? You seem a bit down lately; is there anything you'd like to talk about? Sometimes it can help to talk things over; just know I'm here for you." Explain that sometimes it's easier to frame our problems in terms of food and weight: "It can be easier to count calories than think about how life stinks at the moment" or "Sometimes we think having a certain body shape will solve all of our problems" or "Eating is one way to put off the bad feelings." But also let her know that these are only short-term solutions that won't help with the real issue and can even make things worse. If the issue really is food or weight, ask your teen what's bothering her, why it's bothering her, and what she'd like to change. Ask how you can help. If she's interested in going on a diet, see the advice in Chapter 6. It's important to switch the focus from dieting to healthy weight management, regardless of your teen's weight.

Jack just blew up over the fact that his pants are 1/8 inch too short and said he's not going to the mixer now. Should I leave him alone or say something?

Think about what might really be going on. Is the issue the pants or an overall feeling of social anxiety? Probably the latter, together with fears about an imaginary audience all looking at and talking about his pants. Possible strategies include letting your child blow off some steam without getting too involved (it might just blow over); asking your child what's going on and why he's feeling this way; or sharing a similar experience. Without going overboard about the appearance issues, you can also reassure your child that he looks great and ask him questions to help him realize he's likely being more critical of himself than others may be.

Miguel came home from his first semester at college 20 pounds heavier than when he left home. He keeps patting his stomach and joking about it. I can't help remembering that my own weight problems started when I got to college and stopped growing taller. Should I tell him that so he'll watch it?

First, does the weight gain matter? Miguel may just be experiencing a catch-up weight gain after a late growth spurt. It's important to take into account his overall weight status and pace of physical development. Second, does this weight gain bother Miguel? Although he's joking about it, he may actually be concerned. You can come right out and ask him ("Miguel, I'm wondering how you really feel about gaining weight. Is it bothering you?") or just refrain from joining in the joking. Third, why did he gain weight? Was it due to some underlying stress? Or the result of changes in lifestyle now that he's away from home?

If Miguel's weight gain is due to stress, provide him with the support he needs, encourage him to get support at school if warranted, and explore ways of decreasing stress such as taking fewer classes, decreasing grade expectations a bit, practicing better time management, getting enough sleep, and taking some time-outs for relaxation and physical activity. If Miguel's weight gain seems to be due to lifestyle changes, share your experiences with the transition to college if they seem applicable and help him brainstorm solutions, such as getting up for breakfast to start the day off right, taking advantage of the salad bar at the dorm cafeteria, going to the gym three times a week, or buying a small fridge for his room for keeping fresh veggies and fruit around for late nights. You may want to buy him a book such as *The College Student's Guide to Eating Well on Campus* (see Resources at the end of this book). As much as possible, turn the conversation away from weight . . . and focus on behaviors.

I came home to find Hallie and her friends sitting in the family room surrounded by bags of chips, cookies, and candy—which, they explained, was their "consolation party" after one of the girls had gotten dumped by her boyfriend. I had to bite my tongue to avoid saying anything. Should I have kept my mouth shut?

Definitely. Spoiling their fun would just make you look bad and make your daughter resistant to hearing anything you had to say. You might be able to address the subject later, but it will be hard to do it without sounding critical of the way the girls decided to cope with an unpleasant event. If you can start by complimenting Hallie and her friends for sticking together and supporting each other, you might be able to subtly suggest that they consider a shopping trip for some small luxury or a "victory run" around the park next time. But the most constructive move might simply be to examine the external influences that might have made Hallie think that coping with emotional upheavals by eating was a good idea. Do you console yourself with chocolate after a bad day? You might want to think about alternative coping strategies to role model for your kids. Do you talk about "good" foods and "bad" foods? That type of labeling usually leads naturally to "rewarding" ourselves with "good" foods when we've had a bad day. But do keep things in perspective. A once-in-a-while food consolation isn't going to hurt anyone . . . and it's a lot better than some of the other options.

Jackie, my 13-year-old daughter, made excuses not to be at the dinner table three times last week, and this week it's been four. I know I can't force her to eat, but should I lay down the law about coming to the table?

Let her know she needs to be at the table for dinner with the family unless something special is going on, which she needs to let you know about (see Chapter 11). This is a fair expectation—particularly for a teenager of this age. This will be easier to do if family meals have been the norm in your house over the years. But think about, and perhaps ask your daughter, why she doesn't want to come to the table. Has she just been too busy? Or is she trying to avoid eating? Is the family meal table a place for conflict? Discuss possibilities for decreasing conflict at the dinner table with your teen. "You need to be at the dinner table. It's important to me to share meals with you and hear about your day. Plus, we usually have pretty good food. What's getting in the way of your coming to the table? What would make family meals more enjoyable for you?"

Tamika came home from school in a real funk. I know she must have gotten teased again about her weight, and it kills me to see her suffer like that, but when I try to talk to her, she just gets defensive and shuts me out. What can I do?

First, try to recall exactly what you've said to her. Did you just ask what happened and how she was feeling and then offer your unconditional love and support? Is there any chance that anything you said could have been interpreted as blaming your daughter for being mistreated because whether she's overweight is in her own control? Even if you meant well, if you jumped in and started making suggestions for how she could take off the pounds, you've implied a criticism and reinforced the other kids' right to act on weightism.

Next time this happens, don't offer advice on dieting, changing eating patterns, or increasing physical activity. Instead, listen, be supportive, and let

Tamika know that teasing and other forms of weightism should never be tolerated: "I'm really sorry that happened to you. It is totally unacceptable." Save the advice on eating and activity for another conversation. See Chapter 14 for some ideas on dealing with weight stigmatization.

Eli just came down to dinner and announced defiantly that he had a Polish sausage and a milkshake for lunch with his best friend and doesn't see any point in sticking to something as "pointless" as a kosher diet. This will really bother my parents. What can I say to make him change his mind?

Eating patterns are among the many things that can be influenced by a teen's search for identity, since how and what we eat are integral to how we view ourselves and what we see as important. As teens begin to develop more advanced and critical thinking skills, and progress in their moral development, they may begin to question certain eating patterns. Taking this into account can help you avoid overreacting and lapsing into the authoritarian parenting style mentioned in Chapter 2. In Eli's case, I'd ask why he thinks keeping kosher is pointless. What does he see as some of the advantages and disadvantages? You might even ask him what he would do as a parent in this type of situation. If something is very important to you (such as a diet for religious reasons), let your son know and explain why. Since you probably won't be able to control his eating patterns when he isn't with you, don't even try. But it's fair to demand that certain dietary practices be followed within your home and even within your presence or the presence of others who may find a departure from them disturbing (in this case, his grandparents).

Every day this week I've come home from work to find Andy sprawled out in front of the TV with snack food wrappers nearby. We're already having problems because a couple of times I snapped at him about getting off his butt and he wouldn't speak to me for the rest of the night. How can I get him to see that this is a bad way to spend the time after school?

Probably best not to say anything when you first walk in the house, because it is bound not to be anything very helpful to the situation or your relationship. Find a good time to talk, explore what's going on in Andy's life, and think about a plan with him. If Andy is feeling lonely or bored, show your empathy and explore some options for afterschool activities that he might like to do (for instance, sports, art classes, or a part-time job). Ask what healthier snack foods Andy would like to have around the house, and perhaps go to the supermarket together to buy them. If what's making you angry is having to clean up his mess, make it clear that your son needs to do that himself—just separate that conversation from one about alternatives to unhealthy snacking.

I found laxative packages on the sink in Gabriella's bathroom, and this isn't the first sign she's using them to lose weight. I can't sleep at night, but I'm afraid if I say the wrong thing, I'll never get the truth out of her. I'm so worried!

Here's a case where you can't afford to wait until your teen brings up the topic. If you suspect that your teen is using laxatives or vomiting for weight loss, exercising excessively, or severely restricting her dietary intake, take a deep breath before rushing into things. Don't have the conversation when either you or your teen is rushed. Find a good time and say, " I need to talk with you," or ask your teen if now is a good time: "I need to talk with you. Is this a good time? If not, when would be a good time today?" Plan ahead about what you want to say and decide on the purpose of your conversation—for example, to let your teen know that you're concerned and get your teen to professional help. If you're very nervous about bringing up the topic, do some preparation by writing things down, talking with others, or practicing with a friend or your spouse. Let your teen know you're concerned and mention specific behaviors. "I'm very concerned about you because I heard you vomiting in the bathroom this morning. I'd like to talk with you about what's going on and how you're feeling." Expect denial, anger, or feelings of shame, but know that your teen may also be feeling relief that she's going to get help. Be firm in sticking to the topic and remember your purpose. It's generally better to have a short conversation and leave the door open for further communication than to try to say everything and end up on a bad note. But you may need to insist on professional help, even against your teen's will. See Chapter 15.

Gwen was in the middle of a food binge when I went downstairs at 1:00 A.M. to get a glass of milk to help me sleep. I was so shocked by all the food she'd obviously been eating that I pretended I was too sleepy to notice and hurried back to bed. Then I stayed awake all night worrying about what to do.

Even though you lost a night of sleep (do you know any parents of teens that haven't?), I think you did the right thing in not saying anything on the spot. Your sense of shock combined with her feelings of shame probably wouldn't have led to the most productive conversation. Most people who binge are very much ashamed of their behaviors, so it's extremely important to be sensitive to this in bringing up the topic. Think about how shameful it is to engage in uncontrolled overeating in a world that places so much importance on control and thinness.

Before talking, think about whether this may have been a one-time event or whether you've been noticing other signs of food binges, such as food disappearing or a mess in the kitchen in the morning or when you come home from work. You might say, "I came down the other night for a glass of milk and saw you in the kitchen with a lot of food out. I know that sometimes eating can help take our minds off other problems, so I'm worried about any problems you may be facing. Can we talk a bit?" Be careful about sounding at all judgmental, and, of course, don't say anything like "I'm worried about this leading to weight gain." Keep the discussion focused on feelings and behaviors—not on weight.

Together, you can brainstorm helpful solutions. For example, suggest that when she has the urge to binge, she try to postpone eating by 10 minutes by taking a shower, listening to music, singing a song, meditating, calling a friend, or walking around the block (if it isn't 1:00 A.M.). Sometimes (but not always) the urge to binge will pass. Talk with her about the importance of avoiding long periods of not eating or dieting, since this can lead to overeating; it's better to get into a pattern of three meals a day, with small snacks in between meals. You can also talk about changes that might be helpful at home such as having high-bulk foods such as baby carrots and apples on hand for easy eating. Ask your daughter if there are trigger foods that she would rather you didn't buy and if there are good substitutes that she would like to have around the house. Do *not* avoid buying snack foods altogether or, even worse, lock up or hide foods—even if she asks you to do so. This just plays into making these foods seem like "restricted" or "forbidden" foods, and when she does eat them she will feel even worse about herself. Keep in mind that you can't stop your teen from binge eating, but you should demand that she clean up her mess and replace the food she eats if the amounts are excessive. If this has been an ongoing behavior, I strongly suggest arranging a meeting with a dietitian or a psychologist, since it's very likely that there are some underlying issues that she could benefit from discussing with a professional.

Suki was heartbroken when she didn't get a part in the school musical. We both know she has the best voice in her class, and we both know it's because of her weight . . . the play includes a lot of dancing in skimpy clothes. What could I say that wouldn't humiliate her even more?

First acknowledge how she feels: "I'm sorry. You must be feeling really disappointed." Then try to help her to move from feeling sorry for herself and blaming herself to seeing how the musical is going to lose out and how those who chose the cast are to blame for making a bad decision, "What a loss for them!" You might be able to get Suki to turn her anger into action and go to the musical director and ask on what basis the decision was made, or even go to the school principal. You could suggest this option to her, offer to go with her, or suggest calling yourself, but I don't think I would push this too much. I'm just not sure we're there yet in terms of fighting weightism, and she may end up getting even more hurt.

You could also share this real-life story with her. A friend of mine has a daughter who is a competitive ballet dancer. She auditioned for a number of professional companies and was accepted into most of them. She was not accepted into one, most likely because this company tends to go with long, thin, tall girls and her body type didn't fit this description. Did she complain about her body or go on diet to try to change it? No. She told her mom that the company was stupid to have made that decision because she could dance circles around the girls who did make it. Obviously, this girl has her head screwed on right . . . probably thanks to her mother, who has helped her with self-acceptance.

"Mom, do I look fat in these pants?" When Jasmine asked me that, I didn't know what to say. I thought the pants did look way too tight, but I knew if I said so she'd hear it as my accusing her of being fat. So I said nothing and then spent the evening wondering what kind of mother would let her daughter go out in an outfit that might embarrass her. What can I do next time?

If you really think the pants are too tight, relate your comments to the pants being too tight and not to your daughter being too fat. In fact, it's always best to avoid answering questions such as "Do I look fat?" with "No, you look thin." This can get you nowhere and further reinforces the notion that fat is bad. But you can say something like "It's not a matter of your being too big

. . . but rather the pants being too small. Personally, I don't feel comfortable wearing tight pants. How do *you* feel in them?" Then you might want to suggest a different pair of pants, compliment her on her earrings or hair, and leave the final decision to her. And in answer to your question "What kind of mother would let her daughter go out in an outfit that might embarrass her?" my response is "A mother who understands that teenagers need some guidance but also need to be allowed to make their own decisions and learn from the consequences."

Darryl told me that he wants to start taking protein powder to build up his muscles. I'm concerned about the side effects and tried to tell him what I'd read, but he cut me off with the protest that "a million guys are doing it, and no one has had any problems with it." I'm afraid he's going to do it behind my back if I object too strenuously. What could I say that will convince him he looks great as he is?

Try to find out why he's concerned about his muscles. Has something happened? Did someone say something to him? Take the time to reassure him that he's normal and looks good as is. Talk with him about differences in body shapes and sizes and how different teens develop at different paces. If your son is smaller than his peers, acknowledge that it can be hard, but also look for positive role models in his life that are shorter or thinner than the norm. A former coach? A good friend of the family? Explore alternatives with him such as improving his eating patterns, and ask what you can do to help. Let him know that you're concerned about the protein powders. You can provide him with resources on the topic (see some suggestions at the end of this book) and make an appointment with his physician or with a dietitian to give him an opportunity to discuss the pros and the cons with someone else. Be very cautious about consulting with a personal trainer, a coach, or the person behind the desk at a health food store; they may lack the knowledge and may have vested interests. If your son is involved in a sport, and his coach is against the use of such products (you can call and ask), the coach can be a great resource since coaches can have a huge influence on teens. Your son may decide to go ahead with this plan anyway; if so, don't feel that you need to pay for it, but pay attention to how much of the supplement he is using, whether he is drinking enough, and how he feels. If you have any concerns, arrange for another appointment with his physician.

Juanita came home from school today and told me that she needs to lose some weight—like now! She's planning to go carb-free for the next two weeks and then will start eating "healthy foods." She needs my help in making this happen as her diet calls for things like eggs and sausage for breakfast, tuna for lunch, and either steak, fish, or chicken for dinner. She can snack on things like nuts and cold cuts in between meals. Doesn't sound very healthy to me, but I want to be helpful. What should I do?

First, go back and read Chapter 6 on dieting and Chapter 9 on calories. You'll find lots of the information you need there. Find out why your daughter needs to lose weight so quickly. Did something happen? Is a special event coming up? Regardless of her weight, this is not a good plan. She'll lose weight if she can stick with it, but much of it will be water loss. She's likely to tire of the plan and more likely to progress to binge eating than to "healthy eating." Let her know that you'd like to help her out but want to help her with healthy weight management. Talk about options for modifying her proposed plan by increasing complex carbohydrates to include some whole wheat bread, pasta, and potatoes, but decreasing simple carbohydrates such as those found in soda pop, cake, cookies, and candy. Talk also about the importance of keeping her fat intake at a reasonable level, since fat is high in calories. Explore options for getting more physically active and ask how you can be of help there. Your daughter probably needs some reassurance—be sure to sprinkle some compliments throughout your conversation regarding her appearance, her self-care habits, and her ability to make smart decisions. Don't agree to help her with this diet plan—even for a short period of time. Keep in mind, however, that because she's a teenager, she may decide to go ahead with it. If so, it probably won't last very long, but do keep tabs on the situation. If you're concerned, arrange to have her meet with a dietitian.

Earlier this evening, I heard my daughter Shari say, "Ugh! I feel so fat today. I'm not going anywhere tonight," as she stormed upstairs. Should I call her back down to talk to her?

At some point, every parent of a teenage girl will hear some rendition of "I feel so fat." Our first task in this type of situation is to *find out what's really going on*. As discussed in Chapter 4, fat is not a feeling, so it's important to understand what the real feeling is. Our second task is to *provide our teens with reassurance*. It is best if we can do this without reinforcing the notion that fat is bad and to be avoided at all costs. Thus, while the easiest response is to say, "You're not fat," if at all possible, I recommend trying different responses that provide reassurance. My recommendation would be to wait a while and let Shari calm down. If she is still up her room, go upstairs to talk with her to explore what's going on: "What's going on? What's bothering you? Are you having second thoughts about going out tonight?" If you get some useful information, you may be able to help her sort things out and provide the type of reassurance that is needed: "It sounds like you're a bit nervous about going to the party without any of your really good friends. " Otherwise, go with some general reassurance—"I think you look beautiful" or "You're so outgoing that people at parties seem to like being near you."

Tasha and her friends are sitting at the kitchen table and start talking about which one of them is fatter than the next. I'm not supposed to be listening, but I can't help overhearing. Should I butt in? What can I say that won't relegate me to the ranks of the typical dorky mom?

Since they're in the kitchen, not in your daughter's bedroom with the door closed, I think it's okay to add your two cents' worth—but in a way that won't be perceived as critical or intrusive. If you know your daughter would die of embarrassment if you said anything, or you don't feel comfortable doing so, talk with your daughter later about what you heard and offer some possible alternatives to fat talk. But if you say something to her friends, you get more for your buck: Your daughter hears your message, she sees that her friends approve, and you may have an impact on the teens that surround your daughter. Ask them a question or two: "Why is it that women talk so much about being fat? Who are they comparing themselves to? What does it mean when someone says 'I feel fat'? When someone tells you, 'I'm so fat,' how can you respond without getting down on yourself?"

I really can't win. My daughter complains that she's fat, and when I say she's not, she insists she is fat compared to all her friends. The truth is that most of her friends do happen to be very small and Sophie is 5 feet, 8 inches, muscular, and an athlete. She also happens to be gorgeous, but there ought to be something I can say to reassure her besides the fact that she's physically attractive. What can I say that will make her feel great about herself without reinforcing the "body comparison trap"?

First, acknowledge how hard it can be to feel different—this is where sharing a story about your own adolescent experience, if you have one, can be particularly effective. Then point out role models that have similar body builds. Let her know her strengths will become apparent as she grows older; her peers will look older and, anyway, there will be less need to blend in with the crowd. Encourage her to keep active and remind her to focus on what is controllable; she can control her behaviors, but her body build is not under her control.

Danielle asks me what she could eat that would be "healthy," because she's trying to look her best for the prom that's a month away. What can I say without implying that there are "bad" foods we should all avoid?

Exactly what does she want to accomplish? To lose a couple of pounds? Have shiny hair? Good skin color? Look vibrant? Or all of the above? As always, start by reassuring her that she looks great and emphasize balance: a lot of fruits, vegetables, whole grains, and a moderate amount of dairy foods and meats or meat alternatives. She can go easy on the tip of the pyramid if she's interested in losing a couple of pounds or not gaining weight, but encourage her not to be unduly restrictive, as that can backfire.

Sam has sworn off soda pop ever since his short stint on the cross-country team, when the coach told them how bad it was for runners. Now every once in a while he says he's dying for a root beer. What am I supposed to say about this?

Say, "Then have one." It won't hurt him to have a root beer every once in a while, but he doesn't need soda pop, and avoiding it isn't a sign of an emerging eating disorder. So don't push it if he takes pride in resisting the urge.

Melissa told me she was worried about a friend who admitted to having purged and who already has other problems. When I suggested maybe I should call her father, she made me swear not to. I told her if she was a friend she'd let me do something if such behavior didn't stop right away. She assured me she'd let me know. Was it right for me not to say anything to the girl's father?

This is a tough one. On one hand, your daughter is concerned about her friend. On the other hand, she doesn't want to betray her. Now she's put you in the same bind, but since she's brought up the dilemma, she's looking for your help with a solution. Remind Melissa that her friend may have shared her secret with her because she was also looking for help. Encourage Melissa to talk with her friend and say something like "I've been thinking about what you told me last week. I'm very concerned about you because you told me about your purging. I've also noticed that you've been [name specific behaviors]. I care about you a lot and think you should talk with an adult about this. I'm willing to go with you." If Melissa is strong enough, she can also add, "If you don't do this, I'm going to talk with an adult about it, because I'm really worried." If Melissa doesn't feel comfortable talking with her friend, or talks with her and nothing happens, she should talk with a teacher or social worker at school who can explore the situation a bit more with her friend, without involving Melissa. Another option that Melissa might be open to is having you speak with her friend. The issue of betrayal of trust is important here, but Melissa needs to understand that it's still less important than helping her friend get the help she needs. Whether you should talk to her friend's father depends on so many things that I'd try these approaches first. Whatever you do, *follow up*: Don't forget to ask Melissa down the road whether her friend is still purging, and keep asking if you have any ongoing concerns.

I love my sister, Nancy, but I'm afraid she's undoing all my hard work to make it clear that hurtful weight comments are not acceptable at our home. She's always dieting, and she just doesn't get it. Nancy often comments about other people's weight and provides unsolicited advice to my girls about how much they're eating or "what a difference a weight loss of only five pounds would make." Is there a way to get through to her without starting a family feud?

As hard as it can be to talk with our teens about weight-related topics, it can be even harder to talk about these issues with family and friends. As when talking to your teen, think about the purpose of your conversation and find the right time and place to talk. When you talk, clearly spell out what you're trying to do in your house, without being judgmental, and enlist your relative's support. "Nancy, I'm concerned about the girls worrying too much about their weight, feeling unhappy with how they look, and developing eating problems. So, based on some advice that I read in a book recently, we've decided to stop talking about weight at home. It's really hard, but I can already feel a difference. I need your help with this. I'm not asking you to change your eating style, but I am asking you not to talk about dieting or weight when the girls are around."

In the next chapter, you'll find more tips for dealing with unsolicited advice and comments often made to overweight teens.

"What can we do when problems come up?"

14

Helping Your Overweight Teen
Be Healthy and Happy

*I*f you have a larger-than-average teenager, you may have flipped to this chapter first. The widely publicized dangers of being overweight have made us all consider the subject more urgently than ever. But I hope you'll read much of the rest of this book. The first two sections provide crucial background information on where obesity stands in the full spectrum of weight-related problems and why traditional weight control measures, like dieting, not only fail but may actually lead to disordered eating. The four cornerstones for a healthy weight and body image (Chapter 7) build the foundation for helping your teen. The third and fourth sections provide tips for healthy eating and how to make it happen at home. Thus, this is not a stand-alone chapter, but builds on concepts introduced throughout this book.

By now you know that "going on a diet" is *not* the answer for long-term and healthy weight management. Fortunately, there are effective alternatives for controlling weight. But I firmly believe that goal number one is to help kids accept themselves, *no matter what size body they have.* And even when we get to goal number two, healthy weight management, the aim will be to help your teen take steps to maintain *her* natural best weight, not shed pounds and sculpt her body to conform to some ideal that makes no sense for her.

Fortuitously, self-acceptance may in itself promote successful weight management. In our New Moves program we found that overweight girls who received support and acceptance showed signs of feeling better about themselves and began to take steps toward being more active. Teens who feel better about themselves are also more likely to engage in self-care, including healthy levels of physical activity and healthy dietary practices. And these behaviors stand a fair chance of leading to weight loss, or at least to the prevention of further weight gain, for those who are not already at their natural weight.

what you can do
START BY DETERMINING
WHETHER YOUR TEEN
IS OVERWEIGHT

Weight status is generally assessed by calculating the body mass index (BMI). BMI is calculated by dividing a person's weight (in kilograms) by his or her height (in meters squared). This measurement takes height into account in determining if a person is overweight. For adult populations, individuals with BMI values of 25–30 are considered moderately overweight, and those with BMI values above 30 are considered overweight or obese. Since children and teenagers are still growing, and since boys and girls grow at different rates, it is important to take age and gender into account, in addition to height. Whether or not a child or adolescent is considered overweight is determined primarily by comparisons with reference populations of children of the same height, age, and gender. Basically, children and teenagers who have BMI values above the 85th percentile but lower than the 95th percentile are considered to be "at risk for overweight" or "moderately overweight." Generally, a physician will be concerned about them only if they have other medical symptoms. Children and teenagers who have BMI values above the 95th percentile are considered overweight or obese. Talk to your physician or check out *www.cdc.gov/nccdphp/dnpa/obesity* for more information on determining weight status. Since kids come in different sizes, it's also important to take other factors into account, such as:

1. Has there been a large change in your child's BMI? A large change in percentile, indicating a large weight gain (or loss) relative to changes in height, points to a need for exploration as to what may have caused this change.
2. Are there other health problems that accompany the excess weight such as high blood pressure, high levels of blood lipids, such as cholesterol, and diabetes? If so, this increases a need for weight reduction.
3. A more subjective measure that should be taken into account is the degree to which the excess weight interferes with the child's ability to engage in physical activity. For example, is your teen able to walk

at a moderate speed for a half hour without a feeling of over-exertion? Is your teen able to actively participate in different sports at his current weight? If so, and there are no other health indicators, it may be that your child's weight is a healthy weight for him.

Step 1: Provide Loving Acceptance and Support

When we asked what overweight teens need most to help them with healthy weight management, one of them said, very simply, "The biggest thing is support. We need a lot of support"—a sentiment echoed by many of the others we interviewed. The teens mentioned how important it was to them to be heard and how much they hated hearing "Oh, you shouldn't feel that way" when they expressed their feelings about being overweight. A lot of people who talk to them, they said, just don't *listen* to them. Their words remind us that sometimes we need to refrain from giving advice—and that most certainly includes advice on how to lose weight, which is something they can and do get, unsolicited, from everyone else around them. We need to provide our children with support, listen to what they're saying, and show our love. We can start by understanding what their experience feels like.

KNOW HOW YOUR TEENAGER FEELS ABOUT BEING LARGER THAN THE CULTURAL IDEAL

Don't make assumptions. When you can do so comfortably (see Chapter 13), ask how your teen feels about being larger than her peers. If she doesn't seem inclined to open up, keep your eyes and ears open and create opportunities for listening by going out and doing something together. Here's what we found in our studies:

- **Weight is ranked very high in importance by most teens.** The majority of the overweight teens we interviewed felt that weight was very important, although not the most important thing in their lives. Katie ranked it at about 80 on a scale of 1 to 100, saying that because she was getting ready for college it wasn't her top priority but that it was "up there" and "definitely on my mind." Another girl ranked it as a 7 or 8 on a scale of 1 to 10. Paul, an overweight but very athletic teenage boy, talked about how important it was to "have a good body and not look out of shape or have a gut when you're going swimming and stuff like that." In contrast, Mary said she considered the importance of weight "very low," but she defined that as being bothered about her weight approximately one week out of each month. I don't know about you, but spending a whole week every month feeling bad about how one looks sounds like a lot to me.

• **How your teenager feels about her weight may vary, depending on her age.** Latisha, a high school girl, described just beginning to notice that she was heavier than her peers at around age 12 and not being very happy about it then, but said "You don't really pay attention to it" at that age, as compared with how you feel at 14, 15, or 16, when your response to your own appearance becomes "This is really disgusting!" Her words remind us why it's important to keep addressing body image and weight teasing as our teens get older.

• **Teenagers are proud. The fact that they *say* they don't feel bad about their weight doesn't mean they *feel* okay about it.** Sixteen-year-old Shaundra impressed me with her belief in herself when she said she was always going to walk with her head up, no matter how big she got. This is what we need to promote in our children—a feeling of pride, self-identity, and self-confidence, regardless of their size or shape. But not all teens are that confident. One said that when she looked in the mirror she told herself it didn't matter what other people thought, as long as she liked herself. But she admitted that she often got so disgusted looking at herself that she generally avoided mirrors. Another talked about liking being tall, which on the surface sounded as if she'd found a physical characteristic that she could feel proud of; but then she said that being taller made her feel slimmer because it "stretches it out." Dan talked about having been teased, threatened, and pushed around, and after each of those admissions he made a claim along the lines of "I don't care," concluding with "But that's all right." Is it?

What I took from these interviews was that larger-than-average teenagers are wrestling with how they feel about their weight and how they think they should feel. They're trying to come to terms with not quite "fitting in."

what you can do	Stay alert for statements of positive self-worth and pride, whether tentative or uttered with bravado, and reinforce them. But also listen closely for the self-doubt and the hurt and offer lots of reassurance
REINFORCE YOUR TEEN'S POSITIVE ATTITUDE BUT PAY ATTENTION TO WHAT MAY BE GOING ON BELOW THE SURFACE	

and comfort too. And keep in mind all the other factors in your teen's life *important to self-esteem.* Christine talked about the humiliation of having teenage boys walk up to her and tell her, as a joke, that one of their friends wanted her phone number. Knowing the score, Christine said she just never gives out her number so that no one gets hurt. But such self-protection isn't sufficient. Even when she tries to ignore the individual situations, "so much builds up, and I realize then that they're hurting me."

• **Stereotypes are pervasive—and extreme.** Some of the overweight teens we interviewed talked about assumptions that others make about how much they eat, their abilities to participate in certain physical activities, and even their personal hygiene habits. Be aware that when your teen comes home from school, he may have been exposed to comments such as "He must eat all day long to be that fat!" or "Ewwww, fat people never take a bath!" despite the fact that neither of these accusations is even remotely accurate. One boy painfully reported his peers trying to leave him out of football games and other sports because they assumed he couldn't possibly run. He was constantly forced to challenge them to races to prove he was as fast as, and often faster, than they were.

Thanks to the myth that we can all be physically "perfect" if we just try hard enough, being overweight is often viewed as evidence of a character flaw. Maybe some people assume that anyone who would "allow himself to get fat" doesn't care about personal hygiene either. If we think everyone's natural body size is the same (about a size 4 for girls?), we'd probably naturally assume that larger people can't carry their weight with grace and speed. It's critical that we all do what we can to correct such notions. You can start with your own kids in your own home.

• **Experiences that are unpleasant for most—like having to wear a swimsuit in gym class—can be torture for overweight kids.** The kids we interviewed talked about how swimming, particularly at school in coed physical education classes, was especially hard. They complained about school policies that wouldn't allow them to wear T-shirts over their suits.

what you can do
TAKE STEPS TOWARD MAKING YOUR CHILDREN'S ENVIRONMENT MORE COMFORTABLE FOR TEENS OF DIFFERENT SIZES

Following our interviews, we talked to local physical education teachers and found them more than willing to change their policies and allow the students to wear T-shirts over their swimsuits during class. They hadn't allowed that previously because they felt that the extra material

that can intertwine with her attitudes about her weight to affect
esteem. When other things are going well, your teenager may be
handle being overweight with her self-image intact, but when they
watch out for regression in your teen's development of self-acce
and redouble your support.

KNOW WHAT YOUR TEENAGER MAY BE EXPERIENCING IN A THIN-ORIENTED SOCIETY

• **Virtually all teenagers who are overweight have been subjected t**
some form of weightism. Here are the kinds of mistreatment some of the
teens we interviewed reported:

Being considered unacceptable as a friend. When Clara, an overweight girl,
was new at her high school, she became friends with a girl who hung out with
a crowd of thin girls, who told her she couldn't be seen with Clara because it
would "make her look bad." When Clara said she'd understand if her new
friend went with her other friends, and she did, Clara said she "kind of felt
bad." The look on Clara's face showed she didn't feel just kind of bad, but
very bad.

Being left out. Ever since early elementary school, Amanda said, "I haven't
really had a lot of friends or anything and everyone's made fun of me." Her response was to become depressed and to retreat. Amanda called it "crawling inside myself" and said she "wouldn't let anyone around me find out what was
going on." Another girl described standing around with her non-overweight
friends and being completely ignored when others came up to talk to the
group—as if she were invisible.

Being subjected to verbal abuse and name calling. I'm sure you've heard
these time-honored epithets: Fatso. Tub-o-lard. Fat cow. Pig. Blimp. Contrary
to the old playground defense, names *do* hurt, especially when issued by the
opposite sex. Picture what it's like to be the butt of everyone's jokes, as was
the girl who remembered the other kids trying to exclude her from their jump
rope games and, when she did join in, saying "Oh, that was a 4.0 on the Rich-
ter scale." Sadly, the abuse isn't always limited to verbal attacks. Teenagers remembered being poked, having their hair pulled, being tripped in the hall,
and being pushed around.

Being bullied. One teenage boy talked about how the bullies, who were
taller than he was, would make up a nasty rap about him and sing it on the
bus on the way to and from school.

Being the butt of dating jokes, at a stage of life when sexual attractiveness is

Helping Your Overweight Teen

weighed the students down. We pointed out that other things were weighing on the students' minds even more. This was a nice example of how having an increased awareness to teen issues can make a large difference in the behaviors of other people.

- **Getting new clothes should be fun, but shopping can be a nightmare.** Many of the larger girls talked about their frustration in trying to find stylish clothes suitable for their body shapes and how bad they felt when they couldn't try on the same clothes as their smaller friends or even find anything to try on in the same stores. Clothes used to be made to fit the shape of a person's body, but now it seems we need to shape our bodies to fit the clothes! Couldn't stores benefit from reaching out to the population of teens whose bodies don't fit the norm because they are shorter, taller, or wider than the average kid's? Some ideas that come to mind include having a wider variety of styles and sizes, personnel of different sizes, staff training regarding the needs of customers of different sizes, and on-site alterations. It even seems to me that a successful advertising strategy would be something like "At our store we help you find the clothes to fit your body." Fortunately, we are beginning to see some changes. Stores such as Torrid cater to larger teenage girls and have lots of fun clothes in different sizes.

what you can do
TURN SHOPPING NIGHTMARES INTO ENJOYABLE SHOPPING EXCURSIONS

Planning ahead a bit can help turn shopping nightmares into enjoyable afternoons. Talk with your teen about looking for clothes that suit her and emphasize her positive traits. Call to find out whether stores carry larger sizes, and avoid going near them if they don't. Some larger department stores have personal shopping assistants; you may want to enlist their help if you're taking your teenage daughter shopping for a special event and want to avoid a scene. They can bring clothes from the different departments and have them ready in the dressing room. Ask your teen to invite a friend who is also larger than average, since they can help each other out; the teens we interviewed talked about the importance of being able to get honest feedback from kids their size who understood the issues. Check for stores that cater to larger teens near your home. Torrid's website (*www.torrid.com*) includes a search function that lets you type in your zip code. And when all else fails, you can order directly from the store's website.

• **Jokes and "helpful" remarks can be just as hurtful as direct criticism.** Do you have an aunt, father, or friend who tends to make weight-related comments to you or your children? It's bad enough that our overweight teenagers have to face abuse from classmates and strangers outside your house, but a lot of weight teasing occurs at home. Several girls talked about brothers and cousins calling them "fat horse" or "fat whale." One of them said these comments make her want to stop eating, "to become anorexic and just not eat at all."

WHAT YOU CAN DO TO HELP YOUR OVERWEIGHT TEEN FEEL ACCEPTED AND SUPPORTED

I'm not telling you all this to make you feel worse about your child's plight or to feel pressured to get him to lose weight, but because *I was so struck by these teens' need for acceptance and support from their families and by how much better teens felt about themselves when they got this support*. Here are some ideas for providing the support that your child needs:

• **Avoid weight-related comments.** Pressures to be thin come from everywhere. You don't need to add to them. If *you've* noticed she's gained weight, *she's* noticed, so don't comment on it. Also keep in mind that "jokes" about weight are hardly ever funny, even when made by affectionate family members. Not commenting on weight can be particularly difficult when one parent is thin and has never really had to struggle with weight issues, but the child takes after the other, larger parent. One girl we interviewed actually expressed sympathy for her mother, saying "She didn't expect us to be like this" to excuse the times her mother had said to her something like "It wouldn't be such a bad idea to lose weight." Another talked bitterly about her mother's self-disparaging comments about her own weight, which only seemed to reinforce the idea that the daughter was fat—after all, the daughter was bigger than the mother. See Chapter 3 for ideas on developing awareness of how your attitudes toward weight affect your kids.

• **Counteract the "helpful" comments of others.** Start by addressing the comment immediately with the person who made it, in front of your kids. Keep it brief and to the point, but make sure your child hears you. If your mother comments on your daughter's weight, say something like "Mom, I've just read this book about promoting healthy eating and a positive self-image. Based on what I've read, we've decided to stop talking about weight at home." You can always follow up in more detail later, in private with the person who made the comment and separately with your child. The person who made the comment really might not understand unless you explain why you've decided to take this stand: "Mom, I want to talk with you about what happened before. We're really trying not to comment on weight and appearance any more. It's hard because we're fighting the media and social norms, but I'm convinced that it's important. This doesn't mean that we don't care anymore about eating and weight; we are just trying to do things a little differently. I need your help with this. Okay?" When you talk to your teen, try to give him or her a sense of where the comment may be coming from: "Your grandmother has been on a diet for at least 50 years. I'd love her to change, but I'm not sure it's going to happen. You have my permission to let her know that it bothers you when she comments on her weight, your weight, or Uncle Stan's weight. Otherwise, just try to let it go in one ear and out the other."

You'll have to sense what might work with the people involved. One of my friends, who doesn't like confrontation, has focused on getting her daughters to realize that comments like these are not acceptable and that they should not be taken to heart. She has fostered an environment within her home where her daughters know they're loved, no matter what their size. She does speak with her mother about how hurtful her comments can be, but she's accepted the fact that her mother probably isn't going to change as much as she'd like.

- **Provide support—not advice—in the face of weight mistreatment.** Theresa talked about how friends and family offer true moral support when she's been hurt, telling her not to let it get to her: "We're just there for each other." One teen said her mother's typical reaction was to advise her to "go on a diet and start taking Slim-Fast," a regrettable but understandable response. You may feel pressured to get your kids to lose weight, to prevent them from getting hurt, but leave the advice part for another conversation and react first with unconditional support.

- **Let your teens know you love them and stay connected.** Your teens need to know they have your unconditional love. One girl described her mother as "the type of mom that wants me to be happy," and who backs her up in whatever she's going to do. Beth said her mother had "been there all the way" and would say "It's okay; I love you" when the kids teased her. Pat said, "No one that really cares about me, who truly loves me, talks about me negatively," and this is how Pat described her mother: "My mom loves me. She supports me. She's there for me." Another put it succinctly and in perfect teenspeak terms: "I guess my mom loves me, like, unconditionally."

In a large research study we found that overweight teens who feel more

248 THE FOUR R'S FOR FIGHTING WEIGHT STIGMATIZATION

Dr. Jeffrey Sobal, who has done a lot of work in the area of weight stigmatization, has developed a model that you may find helpful in empowering your teen (and yourself) in addressing weight stigmatization. The model is based on four R's: Recognition, Readiness, Reaction, and Repair:

1. *Recognize* the problem, that being mistreated or joked about because of your weight is as unacceptable as being treated differently because of the color of your skin.

2. *Ready* yourself for stigmatization by strangers, acquaintances, friends, family members, and professionals; each situation may require different responses. Practice responses and try to role-play them with someone you can trust. Sometimes you may choose to prevent being stigmatized by avoiding certain situations that you think will just be too difficult.

3. *React* appropriately to stigmatization to minimize its occurrence and its impact on you. Immediate reactions and longer-term reactions may be needed. In some cases (for example, with family and close friends) this may involve letting people know you find their comments or jokes hurtful. Right away you can say "That really isn't funny. It actually hurts my feelings." Later you can follow up by letting your friends or family know how hard it is to have your weight joked about and that it really is inappropriate. You can ask them not to do it anymore. With others, it may be appropriate to come back with an unexpected response or to ignore the action. Longer-term reactions may include filing a complaint at school and demanding disciplinary action.

4. *Repair* any problems stigmatization may cause. Heal yourself by getting support from family, friends, or a professional. Work to prevent future stigmatization by education and advocacy.

Dr. Sobal suggests using one's hand as a memory tool. The thumb represents stigmas that can be opposed by touching it with your fingers—each of which represents one of the four R's: Recognition, Readiness, Reaction, and Repair.

connected to their parents do better in school and have higher expectations for educational attainment in the future, engage in healthier behaviors such as eating breakfast more often and eating more fruits and vegetables, avoid unhealthy weight control behaviors, and experience lower levels of emotional distress than overweight teens who feel less connected to their parents. From this study we concluded that strong parent–teen relationships can help overweight teens be more resilient to negative stereotyping and discrimination. Letting your teens know you care helps to counteract a multitude of negative social influences.

- **Make sure you give your teens lots of positive feedback about their positive traits.** Some people think that if teens are less satisfied with their bodies, they will be more motivated to be physically active, but in Project EAT we found that, if anything, teens who felt better about their bodies were more likely to be physically active. More important, our words of encouragement help our teens recognize their positive characteristics and give them the strength to succeed in other arenas of their lives.

- **Help your teenager get support and guidance from someone who's been there.** When asked who would be most helpful to them in developing a healthy lifestyle and establishing healthy weight management, many of the teens we talked to said that it could be someone who was not only supportive and empathetic but who knew what it was like to be overweight. One 16-year-old said she thought no one who hadn't been overweight could possibly say "I know how hard this is" with any real understanding. People who've been thin all their lives "just don't get it." Overweight teens want help and support from those "who know exactly how hard it is" because "it's not as easy as some people say."

Unfortunately, I've found that many people who struggle with their own weight are reluctant to offer any advice in this area. They feel uncomfortable in discussing weight management because they're self-conscious or feel they've failed. But it's the shared experience that teenagers want. So, if you haven't struggled with your weight, find your teen an adult who has and who is willing to offer support. Large teens need large role models who've been successful in their lives, who take care of themselves through healthy eating and physical activity, and who exemplify pride in themselves.

WHAT TEENS WANT TO HEAR FROM THOSE WHO HAVE BEEN THERE

If you've ever been overweight, can you help a friend or a student, a niece or nephew, by sharing your experiences and wisdom?

- What kinds of difficult social situations have you experienced, and how did you deal with them?
- What have you learned along the way that has been helpful in   *(cont.)*

both dealing with difficult social and emotional situations and adopting healthy eating and physical activity behaviors?

- What can you do together with the overweight teen to help him and yourself along the way? Can you go for walks together? How about shopping? What about preparing a healthy dinner? How about a discussion on emotional eating? What about some activities in which you can model how it's possible to be successful at different sizes? How about some activities not related to weight, such as career exploration? How about just being there to listen?

In spite of all the weight mistreatment that overweight teens experience in our thin-oriented society, you might be surprised to know that studies do *not* consistently show lower levels of self-esteem among overweight teens as compared to non-overweight teens. Supportive parents, other caring adults, and peers can help in enhancing larger-than-average teens' resiliency. You can make a difference in helping your teen have a positive self-image, and, as discussed below, with healthy weight management.

Step 2: Take Practical Steps to Foster Healthy Weight Management

Helping your overweight teen with weight management is hard. There's no way to mince these words. That's why I wrote this book, and, very likely, why you're reading it. It's hard for you as a parent; you want to help your child lose weight so that he won't have to experience the negative social consequences described earlier in this chapter. You want to protect your child from any harmful physical consequences down the road. Yet your teen, like all teens, is exposed to social pressures to overeat, underexercise, and resort to extreme, yet ineffective, weight control measures when weight problems emerge. And since your teen is a teen, it makes it hard for you to know how to help. No doubt, you've already discovered for yourself that your efforts to help your teen can backfire. The four cornerstones that are outlined in Chapter 7 and elaborated on throughout this book, can be so effective because they allow you to help your teen with healthy weight management in a manner that takes into account your teen's stage of development, particularly his growing sense of autonomy, and his developing, yet still fragile, sense of identity and self-image. No, you can't control what your teen eats, how much he exercises, or, ultimately, how much he weighs. But, as described throughout this book, there is a lot you can do! You can model healthy eating and physical activity behaviors for your teen such as pyramid eating, portion control, and daily physical activity; provide an environment that makes it easy for your teen to adopt these behaviors by having healthy foods readily available, planning family meals, and supporting physical activity; encourage your child to engage in these behaviors which, in the long run, will lead to a weight that is healthy for him; and provide emotional support when your teen experiences the inevitable negative social experiences described earlier in this chapter.

The key is to meet your teen where he is and help him progress from there. Often parents (and health care providers) get in trouble in trying to help children and teenagers with weight management because they fail to meet them where they are with their weight and their desire for change. This is understandable, because as a parent you want to protect your children from the consequences associated with obesity, and you may think your wisdom about this issue should override your son's or daughter's decision making. But in trying to help your child, you need to recognize the importance of readiness for change, to say nothing of preserving your child's self-image and your relationship.

ASSESS YOUR TEEN'S READINESS FOR CHANGE AND MEET HIM WHERE HE IS

Claudia is concerned about her son's weight status. Although she is not overweight, her parents and her brother are overweight and have suffered from some serious cardiovascular problems. She brings her son, Shawn, to see their pediatrician and raises her concerns about her son's weight, particularly in light of their family history. Because of a tight schedule, the pediatrician doesn't take the time to ask Shawn about what is going on in his life, whether he is concerned about his weight, and whether he is interested in making behavioral changes. Instead, he rattles off a list of suggestions: Eat more fruits and vegetables, eat less fast food, drink water or diet pop instead of regular soda pop, and get in at least 30 minutes of physical activity a day. Shawn, who is much less concerned about his weight than his mother is, nods his head while the doctor is talking, but doesn't really take it in. On the way home, he suggests stopping for something to eat. Claudia gets so frustrated when he orders large fries and a milkshake to go with his burger.

Shawn was not yet ready for change. His pediatrician jumped into a behavioral change plan too early in the process. Shawn might have been more successful if his pediatrician had used the time he had with Shawn to find out how things were going in his life, to see whether he was concerned about his weight, and to get a sense of the home environment with regard to eating and activity. He could have let Shawn know that he had some ideas about behavioral changes that don't interfere too much with teen life and kept the door open for further communication. I think it was a great idea for Claudia to take Shawn to see a health care provider. But it might have helped if she had talked to the pediatrician ahead of time, raised her concerns, let the pediatrician know that Shawn was not as concerned about his weight as she was, and asked him how he planned to address the issue with her son. She may have been able to better direct him to meet her son's needs, and he may have set aside more time for their appointment. Or Claudia may have determined that he was not the best choice for her son and looked further for a health care provider who would have taken time to explore Shawn's situation.

In the meantime, Claudia can make some changes in the home food environment such as buying bottled water instead of soda pop, sliced turkey instead of salami, and pretzels instead of potato chips; having dinner on a regular basis; stocking the fridge with fruits, vegetables, and low-fat dairy foods; and making it easier to eat smaller portions by starting off meals with soup or salad and preparing smaller amounts. She can model a physically active lifestyle and provide encouragement and support for Shawn to be more active. In other words, she can work behind the scenes and have quite a big impact in setting the stage for further behavioral change when Shawn is ready.

---

what you can do
WORK BEHIND THE SCENES

Many families get in trouble by trying to control what their overweight children eat. Although such parental intentions are good, this can interfere with a child's ability to self-regulate food intake and pay attention to internal signs of hunger. Work behind the scenes as much as possible by providing adequate support and structure to help your teen make healthy food choices, while avoiding food-related struggles.

Jodi has been gaining weight since puberty. And does it bother her! She's constantly talking with her friends about how fat she feels and experimenting with different diets. After a day or two on the latest diet, or at most a week, she "gives in" and ends up overeating. She gets so down on herself for doing this but just can't stop. Her father, Bill, knows how hard this can be since he's been struggling with his own weight for years. Bill still holds a grudge against his own father, who always made comments about his own weight. So, although Bill would like to help his daughter, he's so afraid to say the wrong thing that he doesn't say anything.

In contrast to Shawn, Jodi is already in the action phase of behavioral change. Jodi needs help in developing a healthier plan for weight management. She could benefit by talking with her father and a health care provider about the importance of focusing on behavior instead of weight and on the value of making gradual changes. She needs information on what is helpful and harmful. She needs a supportive environment. She needs her father to model healthy eating and physical activity behaviors and not diet–binge cycles. Bill may need some help in dealing with his own weight issues. It may be beneficial for Bill to talk openly to Jodi about his desire to help, but also his hesitations in light of what he has gone through with his own weight issues. One of the teenagers we interviewed said parents shouldn't just talk about how healthy food is good for their teens—"they know that"—but rather "show them real-life stuff and talk about these experiences." Bill could say something to Jodi like "I've been hesitant to talk with you about anything having to do with weight because I felt that my father botched it up with me. It's always been most important to me that you feel good about yourself and all your strengths, regardless of your weight. But I've noticed that you're trying different diets and I'm worried about you getting into a pattern of ongoing diets. Over the years I've found it's better to stay away from diets and instead shoot for some changes in what I eat and how active I am. I'd like to help you avoid some of the mistakes I've made along the way. What do you think? How do you think I can help you?"

what you can do

LET YOUR TEEN TAKE THE LEAD IN DECIDING WHAT, WHEN, AND HOW MUCH HE WANTS TO DO

Yes, your teen will make a million mistakes, and you may get some sores on your tongue by biting it to avoid saying things that might not be viewed as particularly helpful. But if you don't let him take the lead, your efforts will be futile.

How ready is your teen to change eating patterns, activity behaviors, or weight status? If your teen is *not yet ready for change*, you can provide an environment that promotes the adoption of healthy behaviors without her even trying. You want your teen to see that it would be feasible and beneficial to make some changes—when ready to do so. If your teen is *starting to think about* weight control behaviors, you want to be prepared to support positive measures when she brings up the topic. Although you shouldn't be taking the lead, your support will definitely be needed to help your teen succeed with healthy weight management. If your teen is *already actively involved in weight control* behaviors, you need to direct her away from unhealthy measures. Talking with an experienced health care provider or joining a supportive teen group can be helpful, and, of course, providing a healthy and supportive environment is essential. Communication is also needed across all three stages of readiness for change, but it can be more direct at the later stages, when your teen is already bringing up the issues. The table beginning on the facing page provides some ideas for meeting your teen where your teen needs to be met.

Some kids may not show any signs of interest in weight control, but parents suspect that their weight is bothering them and that their teens would like to do something about it. If this is the case with your child, arrange to spend some time with your teen—on a walk or bike ride, on a shopping trip, or at a restaurant—and do whatever you can to help him feel comfortable enough to bring up the topic. I truly believe it will come up, but if it doesn't and it's just burning in your mouth, go ahead and bring it up yourself when the setting feels right. See Chapter 13 for ideas on how to bring up sensitive topics.

Other kids may talk a lot about wanting to lose weight, but their behaviors may say otherwise. They may be talking about feeling fat and trying different diets for a day or two, but not making the types of behavioral changes needed for weight management. In this case you might want to encourage your teen to wait to make larger behavioral changes and in the meantime think about what he'd like to change and why. Then the two of you could brainstorm some ideas for very gradual behavioral changes, such as avoiding soda pop, having some vegetables at dinner, or watching a little less television, as well as ideas for making your home environment more conducive to healthy eating and increased physical activity.

MATCHING STRATEGIES FOR HEALTHY WEIGHT MANAGEMENT WITH YOUR CHILD'S READINESS FOR CHANGE

Your teen's readiness for change	Some possible strategies
Low	
• To the best of your knowledge, your teen hasn't seemed to notice or shows no concern about his or her weight.	• First of all, check whether your teen really is overweight. What does your pediatrician say? Does your teen's weight interfere with activities that your teen enjoys doing? If not, there may not be a problem.
• You have not heard your teen talk about any interest in weight control.	• Be glad that your child has a high level of self-acceptance.
• Your teen has not engaged in behavioral changes aimed at weight control.	• But explore a bit further. Look for opportunities to communicate with your teen, so that if there are underlying concerns of which you are not aware, your teen will have the opportunity to discuss them with you. Go shopping together, go out for lunch . . . ask, observe, and LISTEN.
	• Model healthy eating and activity behaviors, in front of your teen when possible. Talk positively about these behaviors (for example, "Even though I am working out an hour every day, I feel like I have more time and energy to do things."). The aim is to get your teen to start thinking about the benefits of making some positive behavioral changes.
	• Does your teen overeat in response to large portions, stress, or loneliness, or to deal with other emotions? Model and talk about responding to internal signs of hunger and satiety and healthier ways of dealing with stress and other difficult emotions.
	• Check out your home environment to see what can be done to make it easier for your teen to make healthy food choices (serve a salad each night), eat regularly (make family meals a priority), and do some family activities that involve action. Through changes in your home environment, your teen will see that it is feasible to make changes—when ready to do so. Through changes in your home environment, you may be able to help your teen make some positive changes without disturbing your teen's sense of self-acceptance.

(cont.)

MATCHING STRATEGIES (*cont.*)

Your teen's readiness for change	Some possible strategies
Moderate • Shows a bit of concern about weight, but it is certainly not the main thing on your teen's mind. • Has expressed some interest in weight control. • May have made some small changes in eating or physical activity behaviors.	• All strategies listed under "Low" are relevant here. However, in addition, you will get an opportunity to respond to your teen when he brings up the topic of weight control. At some point your teen will say something like "I need to lose a few pounds" or "I am starting a diet on Monday." When this happens, consider the following . . . • Put the focus on behavioral change rather than weight. Remind your teen, that if she engages in healthy behaviors, her weight will take care of itself. • Encourage gradual changes in behaviors (for example, cutting down to one soda pop a day, adding 20 minutes of physical activity a day to her routine, or finding an alternative to binge eating when stressed). Your teen will be more likely to succeed in implementing these changes than more drastic changes, and more likely to integrate them into her lifestyle. • Talk about pyramid eating—what it is, why it is important, and how to do it (see Chapter 8). • Talk about nutrient density and the importance of choosing "nutrient-dense" foods (such as yogurt, carrots) instead of "empty-calorie" foods (such as soda, candy) during adolescence when nutrient needs are so high (see Chapters 8 and 9). • When your teen says something like "I want to exercise, but I don't have enough time," use this as an opportunity to discuss time management; encourage your teen to take note of how much time he spends watching television or on the computer (see Chapter 5). • Ask your teen what you can do to be helpful. Make suggestions such as buying certain foods, going grocery shopping together, driving your teen to the gym, or making an appointment with your pediatrician or a dietitian. Make it a priority to follow though in your efforts to be supportive.

- Without pushing too much, ask your teen if she would like to go for a walk with you, go on a bike ride together, or join you at your yoga or aerobics class.

- Provide positive feedback, most of which should focus on behavioral changes rather than on weight.

- This is a good time to provide your teen with some of the recommended resources listed at the end of this book. Some of the teen websites are great. I just love the book *The Right Moves* and the Girl Power website (*www.girlpower.gov/girlarea/bodywise/index.htm*). For older teens, check out *The College Student's Guide to Eating Well on Campus*.

- This is your teen's issue. You are there to provide support, which your teen will need. But avoid getting overinvolved and making your teen's successes and failures your own.

- All of the strategies listed previously are relevant here, but there are two differences: (1) everything is out in the open so you don't need to wonder if you should bring up the topic; (2) your teen is engaging in some unhealthy behaviors and may have some serious underlying concerns that need to be addressed.

- Ask your teen how you can help.

- Take a good, hard look at what is going on in your home. Stop talking about dieting and weight at home. Make weight teasing strictly off limits if you haven't done this already. Make your home a place that does not reinforce social norms regarding the importance of thinness at all costs and in which your teen feels safe from weight stigmatization.

- Double-check and triple-check your own weight-related attitudes and behaviors and identify any areas to be targeted for change. If you feel you can't be objective, ask an honest friend.

- Talk with your teen about difficulties that you have experienced with weight issues. Be honest, but don't feel you need to tell your teen every detail. Remember that your aim is to help your teen. Use that as a guide in deciding what to reveal.

High

- Weight dissatisfaction is very high.

- Sometimes talks about things other than weight control.

- Name the diet—your teen has tried it.

(cont.)

MATCHING STRATEGIES (*cont.*)

Your teen's readiness for change	Some possible strategies
	• Talk with your teen about why dieting doesn't work and how it can lead to binge eating and weight gain. Give her the facts, but try to make it a conversation, rather than a lecture. Do this by asking your teen questions about what she has experienced when dieting. Then reinforce her experiences with research findings (see Chapter 6 on dieting).
	• Talk with your teen about calorie intake versus calorie expenditure, so that your teen will have the know-how to make appropriate choices. Talk about portion sizes and brainstorm ideas for decreasing portion sizes (see Chapter 9 on calories and portion sizes).
	• Encourage your teen to accept the notion that a healthy weight for her may be higher than for her friends. Make sure your teen knows that it is better to be at a higher weight and have good eating and activity behaviors than to be weight cycling and using all kinds of unhealthy weight control behaviors.
	• Arrange for your teen to speak with a health care provider—a pediatrician, psychologist, or dietitian. Do some checking around to make sure your teen will be seeing someone who is sensitive to the needs of overweight teens and will be thinking beyond the goals of weight loss. Work in collaboration with the health care provider to best support your teen. If there is a support group for overweight teens in your community, your teen may find this helpful.
	• Your teen may need some special attention; spend some time with your teen and learn more about your teen's weight worries, body image, and other concerns.
	• Make sure that your teen is aware of your unconditional love—regardless of size or shape.

| **what you can do** | If your child is ready for change, con- |
| CONSIDER PROFESSIONAL HELP | sider consulting a health care pro- |

vider. It's often preferable for some-
one other than a parent to help a teen with the self-monitoring of eating
and activity. Try to find a provider who has experience with teens and is
going to look beyond your teen's weight for success. Start with your pediatrician or family doctor. Or go to the American Dietetic Association's
website—*www.eatright.org*—to find a dietitian near your home who works
in the area of weight management. With all of the attention being paid to
childhood obesity, no doubt more treatment centers and groups for children and teens will be springing up, but currently there aren't as many
good programs around as I would like to see. When you locate one, don't
be afraid to ask questions such as, How do you help children with healthy
weight management without impairing their self-image? Do you put the
kids on a diet or work on a more flexible eating plan? How do you measure and monitor "success"? What is your policy for weighing children? If
you do weigh children, is this done privately?

USE THE SPECTRUM OF WEIGHT-RELATED PROBLEMS
TO TARGET AREAS FOR CHANGE

Overweight teens who engage in unhealthy weight control behaviors are
unlikely to lose weight and may find more success if they stop dieting and
start focusing on pyramid eating (see Chapters 6 and 8). Finding places
where they feel comfortable being physically active may help them feel
better about themselves and their bodies (see Chapter 5). And teens who
feel better about themselves and their bodies may be more likely to take
care of themselves. This is why you should take a look at the spectrum of
eating, activity, and weight concerns discussed in Chapter 1 and see where
your teen is in regard to the different dimensions. Where can you help your
teen move from problematic attitudes and behaviors to healthier ones? For
example, if your teen is not physically active, think about what might be
helpful at her stage of readiness for change. Maybe you need to start just by
making sure she sees you being active and enjoying it. Then you might invite her on a short walk in the evenings. If she seems ready to take action,
see if there's a yoga class at the nearby YMCA or some other opportunity
for exercise where she'd feel comfortable. Let her take the lead and make
the final decisions about what and how much she wants to do, but be there
to support her by being encouraging, giving her a ride to the gym, or paying for a membership at the Y.

what you can do

REMEMBER, THE GOAL IS FOR YOUR TEEN TO SELF-REGULATE HER EATING PATTERNS IN ACCORDANCE WITH INTERNAL SIGNS OF HUNGER

Encourage your teen to listen to her body and pay attention to what it needs. Eating should generally be done in response to physical hunger and not to other internal stimuli (for example, emotional hunger, stress) or external stimuli (for example, large portions, high-fat/sugar foods). Avoid trying to control your teen's intake; she needs to learn to listen to her own body (see Chapters 8 and 9).

LOOK AT THE FACTORS CONTRIBUTING TO YOUR TEEN'S EXCESS WEIGHT

Go back to Chapter 2 and review the possibilities: Is the cause of your child's excess weight primarily genetic? Is your teen sedentary? Does your teen deal with difficult emotions by overeating? Has your teen experienced some type of trauma that has led to overeating? Does your family tend to eat on the run? Is the TV on in your house for more than an hour or two a day? Does your teen's school offer extracurricular activities only to the very fit kids? Does your teen feel uncomfortable in phys ed class? What kind of food is available at school? Are fast-food restaurants lined up on the streets outside your teen's school? Think about what you can do as a family to meet your child's individual needs and to filter out some of the negative influences and reinforce the positive ones.

WHAT A WEIGHT MANAGEMENT PROGRAM WOULD LOOK LIKE IF TEENS DESIGNED IT

We asked teens for their input in designing a program to help them adopt healthy weight management and lifestyle choices. Their feedback has direct implications for teachers and health care providers planning programs within schools, clinics, or community centers. But it's also relevant to parents searching for ways to help their teens with these issues.

The following points are drawn from the teens' responses:

1. Have a leader who understands teens and the difficulties faced by overweight teens. The leader should be able to connect with teens and be encouraging and supportive; outgoing, fun, and personable; willing *(cont.)*

to let participants ease into the program and let students decide what they want from it. If possible, pick someone who has been or is overweight.

2. Provide a supportive, caring, and accepting environment. Teens need to feel comfortable. Provide opportunities to work with others at similar fitness levels.

3. Avoid focusing too much on weight and instead focus on the benefits of a healthy lifestyle. Discuss non-weight-related issues and relate to the participants as teens, not just overweight teens. Include some "teen" activities such as going shopping or having Glamour Shots with other larger teens.

4. Make things fun! Avoid sitting around too much and have lots of physical activity—going for walks in the park, roller-blading, going to the YMCA, playing softball or Frisbee, going shopping together, and having healthy picnics. Sometimes it's easier to talk about feelings while doing other activities: "If it's just sitting down talking, it's sometimes harder to get things out."

5. Include interactive activities aimed at increasing nutritional knowledge and skills such as food tasting, preparation of quick and healthy snacks and meals, making healthy food choices at fast-food restaurants, and identifying low-cost foods that teens like. Have a healthy lunch together "and then talk about what you think of the food."

6. Do whatever you can to make it easy for teens to be physically active and make healthy food choices (for example, have healthy foods available at school and home).

7. Be very sensitive to the issues involved in the social stigma attached to weight in asking teens if they want to participate and in planning activities.

8. Try to reduce the technical barriers often encountered by teens by offering the program at a convenient time, at low or no cost, and by providing transportation if necessary.

9. In determining whether the program worked, don't focus only on weight loss. Look at improvements in self-perception, eating and physical behaviors, and social support. Also provide a way for teens to monitor their progress in achieving their goals.

10. Avoid putting pressure on the teens. Activities should be fun and optional. The teens should have flexibility in deciding what they want from the program.

Reprinted from Neumark-Sztainer D, Story M. Recommendations from overweight youth regarding school-based weight control programs. *Journal of School Health*. 1997; **67**(10): 428–433. Reprinted by permission of the American School Health Association.

Helping Your Overweight Teen

Many people become discouraged when they try to lose weight, get on the scale, and see no change. So put the scale away and measure your teen's success with healthy weight management according to behavior changes like these:

- Your teen feels more comfortable being physically active and tries a new activity.
- Your teen starts paying attention to how much time he spends watching television or being on the computer.
- Your teen gets a passing grade in physical education class.
- Your teen suggests sharing a main dish in a restaurant or choosing the "regular" size instead of the "super" size burger.
- Your teen eats a big salad at dinner.
- Your teen eats only a small piece of dessert.
- Your teen says, "No thanks, I'm full."
- Your teen has a bad day but does something other than binge eat (talks with a friend, goes for a walk, listens to music).
- Your teen feels more pride in herself and starts dressing nicely instead of waiting to lose a few more pounds.

what you can do WHAT TO SAY TO HELP YOUR TEEN SUCCEED WITH HEALTHY WEIGHT MANAGEMENT	What you say during your teen's efforts to lose weight matters a great deal.

To reinforce positive steps, keep your comments positive and focus on behavioral changes rather than weight changes:

- → "I noticed you're eating when hungry and stopping when full. Good for you!"
- → "I think it's wonderful that you're trying new foods."
- → "It's great how you're watching less television and trying to be more active."
- → "'I'm so proud of you for trying out for the volleyball team.'"

When your teen feels as though she has "messed up," remind her that success depends on flexibility:

➡ "There will always be days when we eat more and exercise less. That's normal."
➡ "A real sign of success is following a day when things didn't go as planned with a day of healthy eating and activity."

When your teen feels discouraged about not losing weight, remind your teen to focus on behaviors:

➡ "If you make healthy eating and physical activity choices, your weight will take care of itself."
➡ "Your body may stay at a higher weight than your friends'. But it will become stronger and more shapely, and you will avoid gaining more weight if you keep doing what you're doing."

15

How to Spot the Signs
of an Eating Disorder
and What You Can Do to Help

*H*ave you ever heard someone say, "I'd like to be anorexic for a few weeks" or "I wouldn't mind a bit of bulimia if I could look like [the latest celebrity to be diagnosed]"? I'm always shocked by blithe references that normalize, or even glamorize, anorexia nervosa and bulimia nervosa. Misunderstandings about these serious illnesses still abound, despite volumes of tragic stories about the consequences of underestimating their threat. There are many reasons for the pernicious myths surrounding eating disorders, but it's the product of these fictions that matters most: Failure to recognize the seriousness of these disorders usually leads to a delay in seeking treatment, which has a direct effect on the outlook for recovery.

Make no mistake about it: Eating disorders have far-reaching physical and psychological consequences, and they can take a devastating toll on both the victims and their families. (See Chapter 1 for descriptions of anorexia nervosa, bulimia nervosa, and binge eating disorder.) If you suspect your teen is engaging in extreme disordered eating behaviors, you can't afford to take a wait-and-see attitude. This chapter will help you figure out what to do without losing time worrying about how to approach your teen. If your teen has already been diagnosed, no doubt you've spent many sleepless nights wondering how this could have happened and where it's leading. You've probably felt concern, fear, shame, anger, confusion, sadness, fatigue, frustration, and guilt. The following pages will help you determine how to help a teen who is already in treatment and to get the support you need for yourself. Because it can be so difficult to face the possibility that your teen has an eating disorder, I've included small worksheets for you to record your observations and other material that will help you take action.*

The good news is that treatment can help teens fully recover from eating disorders. Furthermore, treatment can help families improve their patterns of communication and overall functioning and come out ahead. This chapter, which builds on concepts discussed throughout this book, is meant only to give you some background, supportive guidance, and ideas for coping. It is not meant as a substitute for the help of a health care team; *professional help is essential to the care of eating disorders.*

I just don't get it: Why would an otherwise healthy teen do such things?

Why would a seemingly healthy teenager restrict her daily dietary intake to half a bowl of cereal for breakfast, some carrots for lunch, and a salad at dinner; do 5,000 jumping jacks a day; or steal money to buy bags of food, only to make herself vomit after eating it? As hard as it may be to see, eating disorders can serve a purpose:

> Candice moved to a new school when her parents split up last year. She missed her old friends like crazy and had trouble making new ones. What she really wanted was a boyfriend—but no one was looking in her direction. She just felt so lonely in this new setting. On top of the lousy social situation, Candice struggled with her classes. She felt as though her life was just out of her control. Like most teenage girls, Candice reads a lot of teen magazines, where she sees a lot of happy teenage girls with boyfriends—who are, of course, all thin. Candice decided to lose a few pounds, thinking that maybe that would help. Actually, it did help. Candice got so focused on counting calories and watching what she was eating that she didn't have to deal with all those pesky thoughts about her lousy life. Aside from that, she got some compliments from a couple of the popular girls at school, who invited her to sit with them at lunch. They asked her lots of questions about her diet. She decided to keep on going and began restricting what she was eating even more

---

*Throughout this chapter I tend to use the pronoun "she," but the information is just as relevant for boys with eating disorders as it is for girls.

and getting up early in the morning for a run before school. When the feelings of loneliness started creeping back, Candice didn't change her coping strategy but decided to try even harder. She began looking for additional opportunities to get in some physical activity after school, restricting her dietary intake even more, and using laxatives when needed to deal with some eating binges. Now, when Candice's mother approaches her to express concerns about her weight loss, Candice takes it as a compliment. She doesn't see a need for getting treatment—she thinks that these behaviors are working for her and is afraid of letting them go, since it will mean dealing with all of those other emotions.

Candice had a problem, and in the short term the solution she chose seemed to solve it. She was so busy thinking about how many calories were in her food and how she would get out of eating dinner with her mother that she didn't need to think about feeling lonely. And when losing weight helped her fit in at her new school, she thought she must be on the right track. So she kept going and tried harder. Now she greets her mother's announcement that she needs to see a doctor with resistance. But she may be feeling a mixture of fear and relief—fear in that she might have to deal with the original problems and relief that someone is going to help her. Candice's mother needs to know that Candice is likely to be feeling a bit of relief, because Candice is unlikely to show it.

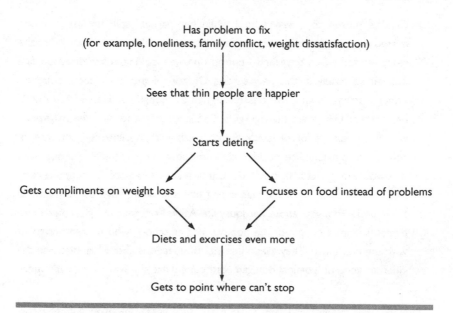

Eating disorders: A solution . . . but the wrong one.

An eating disorder can be viewed as a life preserver; it keeps an individual afloat. A teen with an eating disorder will be reluctant to give up the life preserver until there is an alternative (for example, dry land, swimming skills). I like this analogy, because it shows why an eating disorder might have developed, why a teen just can't stop bingeing or start eating more, why she may deny that a problem exists, and why it is imperative that a teen with an eating disorders get into therapy.

I don't know if my teen has an eating disorder; I just know that something doesn't feel right.

It's not your job to decide whether your teen has an eating disorder. It's your job to (1) identify any possible problems, (2) open the doors for communication with your teen, (3) get your teen to professional help for a diagnosis as early as possible, and (4) work as a collaborative player with members of the health care team if they decide treatment would be helpful.

Diagnosing an eating disorder can be quite complex, even for an experienced clinician. About half of all children and teens with eating disorders don't fit the diagnostic criteria. Teens may have a mixture of anorexic and bulimic behaviors or may meet some but not all of the criteria for a condition. For example, a girl may have all the symptoms of anorexia nervosa but may have lost less weight than listed in the diagnostic criteria or may still be menstruating. That doesn't mean she doesn't need to be treated. On the contrary, she should get into treatment as early as possible since that maximizes her chances of full recovery. Clearly, diagnosis is a job for the best of professionals and not for parents. It's your job to be alert to early symptoms and act to get your teen professional help when you see them.

That's not as easy as it sounds. The power of denial can be very strong when it comes to the people we care about most, particularly in the case of eating disorders. Nourishing your child with food so she'll grow into a healthy adult has been one of your main tasks as a parent. Therefore, it's hard to open your eyes to the signs that your teenager is starving herself, stuffing herself, or purging what she's eating. It doesn't help that we live in a society that practically considers it normal to be dissatisfied with one's body and to diet to lose weight.

If you catch yourself saying things like "Well, yes, her eating patterns have changed, but it doesn't seem that serious. Don't all teenagers go though this type of thing?" get someone else's opinion. Talk with a friend, a school counselor, and/or your pediatrician. If your teen's friends, a school counselor, or someone else raises concerns about your teen's eating behaviors with you, don't dismiss them; they may be able to see things you can't see. Talk with a professional as soon as possible.

So, what should I be looking for?

Some warning signs are listed below. I've broken them up into behaviors, mood, and physical symptoms. In general, you should be looking for behaviors and attitudes that indicate that weight-related issues, eating patterns, and/ or getting enough exercise are becoming primary concerns and are interfering with your teen's mood and involvement in usual activities. Think about whether there has been a *change* in your teen's behaviors (eating, level of activity, social interactions), mood (for instance, she has become more socially withdrawn or lost her spark), or physical appearance (such as weight change).

Behaviors

- Consistently makes excuses to avoid eating meals with the family or engaging in social situations that involve food.
- Has eating rituals to make eating small amounts of food less obvious (for example, cutting food into very small pieces, rearranging food on plate, chewing food a certain number of times).
- May enjoy cooking food for others, but doesn't eat the food she has prepared.
- Has become a vegetarian as another strategy for restricting food.
- Eats a lot of food in response to difficult emotions or social situations (binge eating).
- Exhibits fluctuations in eating—periods of excessive eating cycled with food restrictions.
- Engages in binge eating; you may notice things such as food disappearing, money disappearing (for your teen to buy food), or empty food containers in the garbage.
- Excessive exercising; always looking for an opportunity to be more active, particularly after eating a larger amount of food than usually consumed.
- Exercising without enjoyment; exercise has taken on an obsessive nature and is done regardless of bad weather, illness, or injury.
- Signs of vomiting or laxative use, such as disappearance after eating to go into bathroom, the smell of vomit in the bathroom, or laxative wrappers in the garbage or on the counter.

Mood

- Social withdrawal—your teen is less involved with usual friends and activities, particularly activities involving food (for example, parties, going out to eat).
- Increased difficulty in concentrating, which may lead to homework taking a longer time to complete (and possible decrease in school grades).
- Preoccupation with food, eating, and exercise and continued dissatisfaction with body shape, even after weight loss.
- Just "not the same kid."

Physical Signs

- Weight loss in anorexia nervosa and weight fluctuations in bulimia nervosa (which may or may not be noticeable).
- Coldness, particularly in extremities, which may lead your teen to wear layers of clothing to stay warm and hide a weight loss, even in warm weather.
- In anorexia nervosa, a teen may have increased soft hair on the body (kind of like a baby has—to keep the body warm). There may also be loss of hair on the head..
- Menstrual irregularities.
- Complaints of constipation (asks you to buy laxatives).
- Excessive vomiting will lead to dental problems, and the teen may have a callus on the knuckles from using the hand to induce vomiting.

IS YOUR TEEN DISPLAYING ANY WARNING SIGNS THAT HAVE YOU CONCERNED?

Which, if any, of the signs listed above have you noticed in your teen?

_____

_____

What other signs have you noticed in your teen that have you concerned?

_____

_____

How to Spot the Signs of an Eating Disorder

In going over the preceding list, if you've noticed a few of these warning signs in your teen, you need to think about the next step. You need to talk with your teen in a manner that shows a great deal of caring for your teen, concern about specific behaviors, and firmness about your teen's need for help. This can be a hard conversation to have, and you may be feeling more than a bit nervous in thinking about it. Take a deep breath and think about what you want to get out of your conversation and how best to carry it out. Review Chapter 13 for some tips on communicating with your teen. Remember that your discussion doesn't have to be one conversation; in fact it shouldn't be. But you do need to get the ball rolling. You may find the following points helpful in getting you started:

• *Prepare* for your conversation up front. Write down what you want to say. You may find it useful to practice on someone else. How will you respond if your teen denies the behavior, starts yelling at you, or has some other negative reaction? Other preparation might include finding out about professional resources in your community so you'll have something to present to your teen, talking to teachers and family members in regular contact with your teen to see if they too have concerns, getting advice from friends who have teens to find out how they've addressed tough topics, and reading books like *The Parent's Guide to Childhood Eating Disorders, Surviving an Eating Disorder: Strategies for Family and Friends,* and *Helping Your Child Overcome an Eating Disorder; What You Can Do at Home.* (See Resources at the end of this book.)

• Decide on the *purpose* of your conversation before you begin. What are the main outcomes you want to get from the conversation? Is your goal to express your concern about specific behaviors that you've noticed and open the door for further communication? To get your teen professional help? Know what your aim is so that you can stick with it during the conversation. If your teen tries to get you off-track, you can gently but firmly bring the conversation back to its purpose.

• Choose the *right time and place* for talking. You want to have this conversation when you're feeling semirelaxed and when neither of you is about to go running out or stressed. Resist the urge to bring up the topic when you come into your kitchen and find your teen in the middle of a messy binge or when you're on your way out of the house to make an important meeting at work. Find the right time to talk and place where you can talk privately.

• Talk about *specific behaviors* you've observed. This will make it harder for your teen to deny their occurrence. It's generally better to comment on changes in behaviors and mood than on changes in weight, since your teen may be extremely sensitive to talking about weight and a comment about weight loss that you make with concern may be interpreted as a compliment. Use "I" statements as much as possible to avoid sounding accusatory. Your teen may feel a lot of shame, embarrassment, or fear in being discovered, and it's important to be sensitive to this. Some suggestions:

> "I've noticed that you're exercising more and more lately. Yesterday I saw that you went running before school and after school. I also heard you doing some kind of jumping exercises late at night in your room. I'm worried about how much you're doing and that it has gone past the point of being enjoyable or even healthy. Can we talk about what's going on? Is something bothering you? How are you feeling? What's pushing you?"

> "I'm not sure exactly how to bring this up. Basically, I miss having you at the dinner table with us. Last week you didn't eat dinner with us at all. I want to see what's up and if something is bothering you."

> "A few times this week I've gone into the bathroom and smelled vomit. I also heard you vomiting in the bathroom yesterday after dinner. I'm very worried about you. What's going on? Can we talk a bit?"

> "I found laxative wrappers in the bathroom. I'd like to talk with you about what's going on. Is something bothering you? What can I do to help?"

• *Keep calm* if your teen responds with denial or extreme anger. If she doesn't want to talk, you can say, "We need to talk about this, but we don't need to do it now. Whenever you want, I'm here for you. Let's give it a few days, and then we can talk again." You want to get things out in the open but leave the door open for further conversations. So, it's better to have a short conversation than try to cover everything at once and end up with slammed doors and tears. (And remember, slammed doors and tears happen in the best of families.)

• An important aim of the first conversation, or a follow-up, will probably be to get your teen *professional help*. Your teen may not want to see a health care professional, particularly if she doesn't think she has a problem. Let her know you don't know whether she has a serious problem; you only know she's engaging in some behaviors that are worrying you. A professional can make a more objective assessment. Your teen is likely to be reluctant and may even refuse to see a professional. Is there someone who can help convince your teen of the value of this step? You may need to insist that your child go for help, particularly if her condition seems serious. If you can't get your teen into treatment under any circumstances (and even if you can), go yourself. You'll gain a lot of useful information that will help you help your teen.

EMERGENCY SITUATIONS CALL FOR EMERGENCY RESPONSES

There may be times that you fear for your child's health and safety. If you are really frightened about your teen's condition or have a sinking feeling that your child is in imminent danger, you must take appropriate action and get your child to the doctor's office or the emergency room. You may need to do this even if your teen is resistant to your actions. Let your teen know that you are doing this because you love and care about her and you need to know that she is okay.

Getting professional help: Where do I start? What can I expect?

Start with a family physician or pediatrician. Your child's doctor can do an initial assessment and arrange for your teen to get the additional help she needs. Your child's doctor may stay very involved with the treatment, as the medical director, or may pass your teen on to a different team of eating disorder specialists. This will depend on a number of factors, including your doctor's level of comfort in dealing with eating disorders, the available resources within your community, your child's relationship with your doctor, and the severity of your child's condition.

If you don't have a family doctor, or don't feel totally comfortable with the one you have, talk to people in your area who may have had similar experiences. Or go to the National Eating Disorders Association's website (*www.nationaleatingdisorders.org*) or the Eating Disorder Referral and Information Center's website (*www.edreferral.com*). Both of these websites provide useful tip sheets describing eating disorders and what you can do to help, in addition to information about diagnosis and treatment professionals and facilities. The National Eating Disorders Association's website, as well as the Anna Westin Foundation's website (*www.annawestinfoundation.org*), also provides information on dealing with the insurance aspects of treatment. If your teen is at college, you can contact the college's health service to see if it offers treatment or can arrange for it nearby.

PREPARING TO TALK WITH YOUR TEEN ABOUT BEHAVIORS THAT HAVE YOU WORRIED

What can you do prior to talking with your teen to get prepared?

_____

_____

What do you want to get out of your first conversation (or your next conversation)?

_____

_____

When is a good time to talk?

_____

_____

What are the specific behaviors you want to discuss?

_____

_____

How will you frame your first few sentences?

_____

_____

How might your teen react?

_____

_____

How will you respond? What will you do to stay calm?

_____

_____

What words will you use to get your teen to agree to go to see a health care provider?

_____

_____

Whether your teen will be able to stay at college or needs a break will have to be decided by you, your teen, and a health care provider.

Since eating disorders are complex conditions with medical, psychological, and nutritional aspects, treatment will include medical, psychological, and nutritional components. If you live in a remote area, or if your teen is just showing initial signs of a problem, one or two health care providers may take care of all three of these areas. Ideally, a team of health care professionals, with expertise in each of these areas, will work together. Typically, the treatment team will include a medical doctor, a psychologist and/or psychiatrist, and a dietitian, with others involved as needed. Both individual and family therapy are usually included. Group therapy—teens only, parents only, or teens and parents—may also be included. Treatment options include outpatient, partial hospitalization, and inpatient care. Inpatient treatment will be recommended if your teen's condition is not stable and her health is in imminent danger or if she is not responding to outpatient treatment. Sometimes starting off with inpatient treatment may be recommended to get the ball rolling.

It's important to prepare yourself for a long haul, although this may not be necessary if you're lucky and if treatment begins early. All your teen may need are a few meetings with a dietitian to help her better plan her eating patterns or with a psychologist to discuss some difficulties she's been facing in school. Treatment is often longer, however, and it's important to stick with it. If you feel progress is insufficient, honestly raise your concerns with the health care team. Sometimes a change in providers will be needed. When things are getting you down, remember that treatment takes a while—but it works. Your teen, and your family, may emerge stronger, happier, and healthier.

Where do I fit into the treatment process?

It's important that you get your own needs met and questions answered while also preserving your child's right to confidentiality. This can be very tricky, and parents sometimes feel as if they're being pushed out of the picture. It's hard to feel you're being told to "stay out of it" while you're watching your child suffer; even worse to feel blamed for your child's problem. Up front, I suggest raising these issues with the health care team and coming to some sort of acceptable arrangement. Ask, "How will we, as parents, be kept in the picture? What should I do if I have specific questions? What do I do if I see that my child isn't following through on the treatment plan? What do I do if I see that my child isn't eating? How much can I talk to my child about what she is doing in therapy? How can I get the support I need?"

Pressuring your teen to change her eating patterns may be counterproductive to your teen's progress and to your relationship. Since issues of appropriate boundaries, control, and autonomy are central to recovery from eating disorders, it's particularly important for you to let your teen work with the health care team without interfering. On the other hand, you need to have a sense of the major issues and how treatment is progressing. You need to have your questions answered. And you need to know what you should be doing to help your teen—and not only what you should *not* be doing. Ideally, the treatment process should allow the health care providers to take care of the eating disorder and permit you to focus on your relationship with your teen.

Your role in helping your teen recover is absolutely essential. The health care team needs you to provide your teen with a loving home in which firm boundaries are established. In fact, one of the key tasks facing eating disorder professionals is to help parents get back into the driver's seat and feel empowered to act as the parents their teens need. When you have doubts about fulfilling this responsibility, maybe you can keep in mind a vision that has remained with me ever since we treated a particular teen for eating disorders many years ago. She described how great it was for her to go on a family trip because her parents sat in the front seat and the kids sat in the back. This provided her with a feeling of security. This vision has often guided me as a parent. I take note of who is in the driver's seat, and when I realize that it's one of my children instead of one of the parents, I know something needs to change. Think about your own family. Based on this analogy, where do you see each family member in the car? Are you happy with the configuration? If not, what would you like it to be? What are some steps you can take to make this happen?

If family is so important to recovery, doesn't that mean that we're also to blame?

It's highly likely that you're asking yourself if you're to blame for your teen's eating problems. You may be going over and over scenes in your head and thinking, "What did we do wrong? What could we have done differently?" I urge you to go back to Chapter 2 to remind yourself about the many factors that contribute to the onset of a weight-related problem. Family is one layer of influence . . . but there are many others. Sure, you've made mistakes along the way. Who hasn't? But I imagine that you tried your hardest and did your best, given the circumstances. I urge you to reframe your wonderings into questions such as "What can we do differently now? As a family, how can we best help our child, given her individual characteristics and her social environment? How can we best work to counteract harmful influences and reinforce positive influences?" This will be much more effective in helping your teen recover and in helping your family function even better than it did before.

Use this as an opportunity to look forward and move forward. Try to avoid getting into the blame game with yourself or other family members. Try telling yourself and others things such as "Well, we've made some mistakes, but who hasn't? We're looking forward now and thinking how to make our home one in which everyone feels comfortable, regardless of his or her size. We're looking for ways to really talk with each other about what's going on in our lives. We're using this as an opportunity for growth."

It's hard not to blame yourself when other people (particularly parents of children who appear to be "perfect") make comments about "those parents who don't spend enough quality time with their kids" or about "how they never let their children watch television or eat junk food." (Honestly, don't you just want to slug them?) But you have a lot of work to do now and don't have extra time or energy to waste by ruminating about what you should have done. Now is the time to look ahead and think about how best to meet your child's needs and how to counteract harmful influences and reinforce positive influences in your teen's life.

Is your health care team supporting you in doing these things? If it's treating you as the problem instead of helping you become part of the solution, raise your concerns. You may be able to find a better way to work together to meet your teen's needs.

What about me? What about the rest of my family?

Having a child with an eating disorder can be draining, for you and for your entire family. Some families come through crises ahead of where they started. In part, this depends on where they were to begin with. But it also depends on how they deal with the crisis. Your child needs you. At some level, this eating disorder may be a cry for help. You will need to make taking care of your child a top priority. But you will not be able to do this on an empty tank of gas. You need to refuel your own energy by getting enough sleep, having some relaxation time, having some fun time with your family and friends, talking about topics other than your teen's eating disorder, and having some time to do the things you like to do.

Besides the support you have a right to expect from the health care team, the support of family and friends can make a difference. Also get support from parents of teens with eating disorders, with both the practical issues, such as how to handle insurance problems, and the emotional ones—the pain you're feeling, the sense of loss, fears for the future, keeping up hope, and coping strategies. All parents involved in caring for your child (such as stepparents living in the home, a parent who doesn't live at home) should, ideally, participate in a parent group. If you're lucky, a parent group will be associated with your teen's treatment center. If not, you'll need to look for another type of support group or develop your own network via telephone, e-mail, or, preferably, in person.

At a recent conference of the National Eating Disorders Association that I attended, Dr. Ellen Kerber (a family physician), Kitty Westin (a mother of a daughter who had anorexia nervosa), and Joe Kelly (an author of books for fathers of daughters) presented a model for organizing a family support group for families affected by an eating disorder, Helping and Healing Ourselves. They've developed some guidelines for a meeting format, ground rules, and topics for discussion, including the costs of the illness to the family, self-care, sadness and dealing with lost dreams, appreciation of good days, and hope and comfort. Check the Anna Westin Foundation website for more information (*www.annawestinfoundation.org*).

EATING DISORDERS AND DIABETES

In a large research study, we found that teens with different types of chronic physical conditions are more likely to engage in disordered eating behaviors than other teens. Much of the research exploring the connections between physical conditions and eating disorders has focused on eating disorders among youth with diabetes. Teens with diabetes need to pay a lot of attention to what they are eating, and this may place them at risk for eating problems. Furthermore, teens with Type 1 diabetes often have better regulation when they're at a slightly higher body weight than their peers, which they may find disturbing in light of our societal emphasis on thinness. Finally, teens receiving insulin have their own method for weight regulation: They can take less insulin than prescribed, which can have detrimental effects on their bodies. As a parent of a teen with diabetes, you will need to take extra care within your home to put the emphasis on eating and regulating weight for health—and not to achieve a body shape that is considered beautiful by our culture. If you see any signs of an eating disorder, talk to your teen's diabetes health care team as soon as possible.

EATING DISORDERS DON'T ALWAYS OCCUR ON THEIR OWN

Sometimes teens with eating disorders will experience other emotional disturbances or behavioral problems. An underlying disturbance can lead to more than one problem. For example, a tendency toward impulsivity may lead to both bulimia nervosa and substance use. Or one problem may lead to another. For example, depression may express itself as an eating disorder within a society that places so much emphasis on body shape and weight. Or teens in recovery from substance use may turn to food for comfort or develop other food-related problems. Depending on the severity of the coexisting conditions, your health care provider may decide to treat one before the other.

Boys and Eating Disorders

If your son has an eating disorder, you may be facing additional challenges above and beyond those faced by parents of girls with eating disorders, related to (1) a delayed diagnosis of the eating disorder, (2) the stigma associated with regarding an eating disorder as a "girl's disease," and (3) increased difficulty in finding formal support networks for treatment and informal support networks for him and for you.

If you see any warning signs of an eating disorder in your son, you will have to work extra hard not to push them aside and not to listen to those who don't believe that boys can have these illnesses in the first place. You will need to look a bit harder to find a suitable health care provider who knows that boys do get eating disorders and knows how to treat them, although it's not as difficult as it used to be. You may also need to work harder to get both your son and you the necessary support.

Because it's true that homosexual males and boys who have experienced sexual or physical abuse are more likely than other boys to engage in disordered eating behaviors, I urge you to be open to these possibilities and explore them with your son and his health care team. But you also need to know that the majority of young men who develop eating disorders are heterosexual and have not been sexually abused. As is the case with girls, eating disorders in boys are caused by an array of individual, familial, peer, school, community, and societal factors (see Chapter 2). But you may need to debunk any myths regarding eating disorders among boys that come in the form of comments that make you and your son feel uncomfortable.

WORDS TO REMEMBER FROM EATING DISORDER PROFESSIONALS ACROSS THE WORLD

In the course of writing this book I have visited eating disorder clinics throughout the world. Their professionals offer the following words of wisdom for parents:

- Recognize the power of denial. If you suspect eating disorder symptoms, get an objective health care professional involved as early as possible.

- Take a good look at your own attitudes and behaviors (see Chapter 3). Are you eating only low-fat foods? Are you afraid of your teen's gaining weight? You will need to deal with these concerns and make some changes.

- Don't get tied up in feelings of blame; look forward to what you can do now. Remember that no one person is responsible for the eating disorder, but everyone needs to take responsibility for helping the child get better.

- Be strong in enforcing rules set by your health care team. Your child needs you to be a parent now more than ever.

- Leave the eating disorder to the professionals. You take care of your child. Find things to do with your child that both of you enjoy doing— and do them.

- Work with the professionals. Talk with them about your concerns about the treatment plan, about your teen's progress, and about difficulties you're facing. Ask them what you can be doing to help your child.

- Look for ways to communicate with your child—at family meals, in the car, and at any other opportunity.

- Treatment can take a long time; stick with it.

- Get support for yourself as a parent. Find a supportive group of parents whose children have similar problems.

- Don't give up hope. Treatment can be very successful, and your support will make a big difference.

- Let your children know that you love them … even, or especially, when they seem as though they don't want or need your love. Do this with words, touching, notes, acts of kindness, and through giving your time.

At one of the eating disorder clinics I visited in Israel while writing this book, I received an important piece of advice from one of the staff members: "Parents do not have the right to give up on hope for their child." This is a pretty strong statement, but it's one to keep in mind. Recovering from an eating disorder can be a long haul. But with early intervention, strong parental support, and the involvement of an experienced health care team, your teen's chances for recovery are excellent.

Furthermore, as a result of a lot of introspection, on your own and with the help of a professional team, you may find yourself strengthened—as a person, a parent, and a family. You will probably learn to modify your expectations of others, particularly your children. (An expression I learned about teens, which I love, is that "expectations are premeditated resentments," so it's a good idea not to have too many of them.) You will learn to focus on what you can control (your own behaviors) and not try to control other people's behaviors (including your children's behaviors). You may find that patterns of communication within your family improve and that you learn to resolve conflict in more meaningful ways than you did in the past. You may find new friends along the way who are facing similar challenges and develop strong bonds with them. You will, I hope, adopt some of the key principles discussed throughout this book: modeling behaviors you want your children to adopt, focusing on behaviors and not on weight, making your home environment one in which healthy choices are the easy choices, and providing a supportive environment in which your teens feel accepted and loved, regardless of their size. Through all this, you will help your children to function in a world in which fat is pushed and thin is rewarded. You will help your teens care about eating, activity, and weight . . . but not too much.

Resources for Parents and Teens

Books for Parents

The following are some books for parents on raising teens, helping teens in the prevention and treatment of eating and weight problems, and taking care of your own eating, activity, and weight concerns:

Body Aloud! Helping Children and Teens Find their Own Solutions to Eating and Body Image by Elizabeth Scott and Connie Sobczak. Berkeley, CA: Body Positive, 2002 (Phone: 510-548-0101; e-mail: *bodypos@lmi.net*; website: *www.thebodypositive.org*).—This is a guidebook for parents, teachers, and other adults interested in helping girls (or could be adapted for boys) develop a youth-led program in their schools or youth organizations to promote size acceptance and leadership skills and prevent eating disorders.

Bodylove: Learning to Like Our Looks and Ourselves: A Practical Guide for Women by Rita Freedman. Carlsbad, CA: Gurze Books, 2002.—Techniques and exercises women can use to become less critical of their own physical appearance.

Body Thieves: Help Girls Reclaim Their Natural Bodies and Become Physically Active by Sandra Friedman. Vancouver, Canada: Salal Books, 2002.—Offers strategies for parents, educators, and professionals to help girls deal with excessive societal pressures to be thin and to help them find their voices and identify their true feelings.

Body Wars: Making Peace with Women's Bodies by Margo Maine. Carlsbad, CA: Gurze Books, 1999.—An activist guide to help children and adults feel comfortable in their bodies.

The BodyWise Woman by Judy Mahle Luttter and Lynn Jaffee. Champaign, IL: Human

Kinetics, 1996. (website: *www.humankinetics.com*).—An informative and motivational book about physical activity in women. The book also includes a chapter on getting your children to be active.

Caring for Your Teenager by the American Academy of Pediatrics with Donald E. Greydanus and Philip Bashe. New York: Bantam Dell, 2003.—Comprehensive, informative, and user-friendly guide to parenting young adults through transitions from 12 to 21 years.

Children and Teens Afraid to Eat: Helping Youth in Today's Weight-Obsessed World by Frances M. Berg. Hettinger, ND: Healthy Weight Network, 2001.—Explains how parents, counselors, teachers, and friends can help adolescents challenge social pressures to be thin.

Father Hunger: Fathers, Daughters and Food by Margo Maine. Carlsbad, CA: Gurze Books, 2004.—A description of the important role that fathers play in their daughters' lives.

Fat Talk: What Girls and Their Parents Say about Dieting by Mimi Nichter. Cambridge, MA: Harvard University Press, 2000.—A description of a large research study that explored how teenage girls talk about their bodies and their dieting behaviors, with some great quotes and good advice based on the findings. Includes a chapter on looking good among African American girls.

Great Shape: The First Fitness Guide for Large Women by Pat Lyons and Debby Burgard. Lincoln, NE: iUniverse.com, 2000.—A guidebook promoting physical activity at all sizes.

Helping Your Child Lose Weight the Healthy Way: A Family Approach to Weight Control by Judith Levine and Linda Bine. New York: Citadel Press, 2001.—A guide for parents of overweight children and adolescents, ages 2–18, who are interested in helping their children lose weight.

Helping Your Child Overcome an Eating Disorder: What You Can Do At Home by Bethany A. Teachman, Marlene B. Schwartz, Bonnie S. Gordic, and Brenda S. Coyle. Oakland, CA: New Harbinger, 2003.—Guide and workbook for parents of children with eating disorders.

How Did This Happen?: A Practical Guide to Understanding Eating Disorders—for Teachers, Parents, and Coaches by the Institute for Research and Education. Carlsbad, CA: Gurze Books, 1999.—Helpful tips for parents, teachers, and coaches to support youth with eating disorders.

How to Get Your Kid to Eat ... But Not Too Much by Ellyn Satter. Boulder, CO: Bull Publishing, 1987 (website: *www.ellynsatter.com*).—Provides parents with simple ground rules for promoting the development of healthy eating habits in children.

Overcoming Overeating by Jane R. Hirschman and Carol H. Munter. New York: Ballantine Books, 1988.—A plan for breaking out of the diet–binge cycle.

A Parent's Guide to the Teen Years: Raising your 11- to 14-Year-Old in the Age of Chat Rooms and Navel Rings by Susan Panzarine. New York: Facts on File, 2000.—A guidebook for parents of young adolescents that touches on different aspects of adolescent development and how best to address the needs of teenagers.

The Parents' Guide to Childhood Eating Disorders: A Nutritional Approach to Solving Eating Disorders by Marcia Herrin and Nancy Matsumoto. New York: Holt, 2002.— Guide for parents including information on spotting early warning signs, normalizing eating and exercise, dealing with school, friends, sports, knowing when to seek professional help, and avoiding a relapse.

Secrets of Feeding a Healthy Family by Ellyn Satter. Madison, WI: Kelcy Press, 1999.— Guide for parents who want to foster good health and good eating habits in their home. Includes some easy meal planning ideas and recipes.

Surviving an Eating Disorder: Strategies for Family and Friends by Michele Siegel, Judith Brisman, and Margo Weinshel. New York: HarperCollins, 1997.—Excellent resource for family members and friends of an individual with an eating disorder.

Underage and Overweight: America's Childhood Obesity Crisis—What Every Family Needs to Know by Frances Berg. Long Island City, NY: Hatherleigh Press, 2004.—A description of the problem of obesity among youth and suggestions for families, schools, and health care providers using a paradigm that aims to normalize eating and physical activity.

When Girls Feel Fat: Helping Girls through Adolescence by Sandra Friedman. Westport, CT: Firefly Books, 2000.—Advice for parents, educators, and other professionals on female development, the promotion of a healthy body image and self-esteem, and the prevention of eating disorders.

When Your Child Has an Eating Disorder: A Step-by-Step Workbook for Parents and Caregivers by Abigail H Natenshon. Carlsbad, CA: Gurze Books, 1999.—A guide for parents seeking to assist their adolescent in recovering from an eating disorder.

Your Dieting Daughter: Is She Dying for Attention? by Carolyn Costin. New York: Brunner/ Mazel, 1996.—A very thoughtful and informative book for parents of girls who display early signs of an eating disorder or who have been diagnosed with an eating disorder.

On-Line Resources for Parents

See the following on-line resources for information on eating, activity, and weight (see also the websites for organizations).

Boasting Body Image at Any Weight
Information on activism, ideas for enhancing body image, and a variety of resources. Includes links to other interesting sites. Appropriate for parents and teens.

Website: *www.bodypositive.com*

Centers for Disease Control and Prevention: Overweight and Obesity

Information on Body Mass Index calculation, determination of weight status, and general guidelines and resources. Includes links to many other sites.

Website: *www.cdc.gov/nccdphp/dnpa/obesity*

Perfect Illusions: Eating Disorders and the Family

Information, resources, and a documentary that explores the role of families in eating disorders.

Website: *www.pbs.org/perfectillusions*

Ready Set Go

Tips and advice for parents to promote physical activity in youth.

Website: *www.readysetgo.org*

Something Fishy: Webset on Eating Disorders

Information on eating disorders and chat room support groups for individuals with eating disorders and their loved ones.

Website: *www.somethingfishy.org*

Stop Commercial Exploitation of Children (SCEC)

Find opportunities for advocacy, an informational newsletter, and useful links at the site of this coalition working to protect children and adolescents from the effects of commercial marketing.

Website: *www.commercialexploitation.com*

Weight-control Information Network (WIN): Helping Your Overweight Child

Strategies for parenting an overweight child and supporting healthy eating and physical activity.

Website: *www.win.niddk.nih.gov/index.htm*

VERB—Parents

Ideas and strategies to help parents promote physical activity in preadolescent children.

Website: *www.verbparents.com*

Books and Magazines for Teens

The following are books and magazines for teens on adolescent development, healthy eating and physical activity, self-image, and eating disorders.

The Beginner's Guide to Eating Disorders Recovery by Nancy J. Kolodny. Carlsbad, CA: Gurze Books, 2004.—A guide for teens and young adults who have eating disorders and their loved ones.

The College Student's Guide to Eating Well on Campus by Ann Selkowitz Litt. Bethesda, MD: Tulip Hill Press, 2000.—Candid nutrition advice, facts on eating disorders and substance use, and simple recipes for college students. Excellent gift for a teenager going off to college.

Eating Disorders: A Handbook for Teens, Families and Teachers by Tania Heller. Jefferson, NC: McFarland, 2003.—Provides facts on eating disorders, warning signs, complications, and information on both treatment and prevention. Includes a chapter on eating disorders in males.

Fitness Training for Girls: A Teen Girls' Guide to Resistance Training, Cardiovascular Conditioning and Nutrition by Katrina Gaede, Alan Lachica, and Doug Werner. San Diego, CA: Tracks Publishing, 2001.—This book can guide teenage girls interested in developing a serious fitness training plan. Includes details on resistance training and weight lifting.

Food Fight: A Guide to Eating Disorders for Preteens and Their Parents by Janet Bode. New York: Alladin Paperbacks, 1997.—Includes separate sections for younger teens who are struggling with eating disorders and for their parents.

Fueling the Teen Machine by Ellen Shanley and Colleen Thompson. Boulder, CO: Bull Publishing, 2001.—Recipes and practical information for teens on a range of nutrition topics, including the Food Guide Pyramid, weight management, eating disorders, vegetarianism, and fast food.

Girl Power in the Mirror by Helen Cordes. Minneapolis, MN: Lerner, 1999.—Resource for young adolescent girls on body image, self-confidence, and inner beauty.

Got It Goin' On–II: Power Tools for Girls by Janice Ferebee. Washington, DC: Got It Goin' On, 2000 (website: *www.janiceferebee.com*).—A book for 12- to 17-year-old girls aimed at promoting a positive self-image, spiritual grounding, and healthy lifestyle choices. The book is particularly targeted at girls of color.

Growing and Changing: A Handbook for Pre-Teens by Kathy McCoy and Charles Wibblesman. New York: Perigee Books, 2003.—Answers for youth in the transition to adolescence on body image, eating disorders, fitness, and more.

The Healthy College Cookbook by Alexandra Nimetz, Jason Stanley, and Emeline Starr. New York: Storey Books, 1999.—A collection of simple recipes written by college students for college students. I might steal some of these for quick dinner ideas.

New Moon: The Magazine for Girls and their Dreams. New Moon Publishing, P.O. Box 3587, Duluth, MN 55803-3587; website: *www.newmoon.org.*—A magazine for 8- to 14-year-old girls that focuses on accomplishments of girls that are not appearance-related.

No Body's Perfect: Stories by Teens about Body Image, Self-Acceptance, and the Search for Identity by Kimberly Kirberger. New York: Scholastic, 2003.—Stories and poems from real teens along with personal tales and advice from the author to help girls appreciate themselves.

Nutrition for health, Fitness, and Sport by Melvin H. Williams. New York: McGraw-Hill, 1999.—A comprehensive book on nutrition and sports. This book is meant to be used as a college textbook, but I include it here as a reference for older teens and their parents.

Over It: A Teen's Guide to Getting Beyond Obsession with Food and Weight by Carol Normandi and Laurelee Roark. Novato, CA: New World Library, 2001.—Guides readers toward a deeper understanding of their feelings and a healthier self-image.

PERK!: The Story of a Teenager with Bulimia by Liza F. Hall. Carlsbad, CA: Gurze Books, 1997.—A novel about one young woman's struggle with bulimia for teens who want to understand eating disorders for their own sake or to help a friend.

Real Girl Real World: Tools for Finding Your True Self by Heather Gray and Samantha Phillips. Seattle, WA: Seal Press, 1998.—Encourages young women to be their own persons. Explores beauty standards, body image, eating disorders, sexuality, and feminism through personal narratives.

The Right Moves: A Girl's Guide to Getting Fit and Feeling Good by Tina Schager and Michel Schuerger. Minneapolis, MN: Free Spirit, 1998.—An informative, but fun and easy-to-read book for teenage girls aimed at promoting self-esteem, healthy eating patterns (including vegetarianism), and physical activity.

Taking Charge of my Mind and Body: A Girl's Guide to Outsmarting Alcohol, Drug, Smoking, and Eating Problems by Gladys Folkers and Jeanne Engelman. Minneapolis, MN: Free Spirit, 1997.—A book for girls aimed at helping them to make smart decisions to become better communicators, build stronger relationships, and take care of their physical and mental health.

The Teenage Body Book by Kathy McCoy and Charles Wibbelsman. New York: Berkley, 1999.—A comprehensive guide for teens about physical and emotional development and health issues of relevance to teens such as puberty, sexuality, substance use, stress, eating, and physical activity.

Teen Voices. P.O. Box 120027, Boston, MA 02110-0027; phone: 888-882-TEEN; website: *www.teenvoices.com.*—A feministic magazine for older teens in which articles are written by and for teenage girls.

Vegetables Rock!: A Complete Guide for Teenage Vegetarians by Stephanie Pierson. New York: Bantam Books, 1999.—Written by the mother of a teenage vegetarian, this book includes nutrition information for teenage vegetarians and their parents, ideas for eating out, cooking tips, and 60 basic recipes.

Vegetarianism for Teens by Jane Duden. Mankato, MN: Capstone Press, 2001.—Colorful book with basic information for younger teens on vegetarianism—definition, historical information, nutrition information, meal planning, eating out tips, and glossary.

The Vegetarian Manifesto by Cheryl L. Perry, Leslie A. Lytle, and Theresa Jacobs. Philadelphia: Running Press, 2004.—A handbook for teenage vegetarians that uses data from teen web chat groups, interviews, and focus groups and presents useful advice on nutrition basics and maintaining a healthy weight.

When Dieting Becomes Dangerous: A Guide to Understanding and Treating Anorexia and Bulimia by Deborah M. Michel and Susan G. Willard. New Haven, CT: Yale University Press, 2003.—An informative book about eating disorders, why they happen, and their treatment, for older adolescents and their loved ones.

On-Line Resources for Teens

Clueless in the Mall (Texas A&M University)
Interactive site designed to teach adolescents about eating foods rich in calcium for bone health.

Website: *calcium.tamu.edu*

Do You Have a Smart Mouth? (Center for Science in the Public Interest)
Interactive site with messages about the influence of industry on food choice and healthy eating.

Website: *www.cspinet.org/smartmouth*

Girl Power: Body Wise
Facts on body image, eating disorders, feeling fit, eating right, and growing up.

Website: *www.girlpower.gov/girlarea/bodywise/index.htm*

Health Finder for Teenagers (U.S. Department of Health & Human Services)
Search engine with reliable health information for teens on eating disorders, nutrition, and exercise.

Website: *www.healthfinder.gov/justforyou*

The Melpomene Institute for Women's Health Research—GIRLWISE
A resource for adolescent girls that includes information on self-esteem, physical activity, nutrition, body image, mental health, and more.

Website: *www.melpomene.org/girlwise/girlwise.htm*

The Nemours Foundation

Educational information on food, fitness, and eating disorders.

Website: *www.nemours.org* or *www.teenshealth.org*

Powerful Girls Have Powerful Bones (Centers for Disease Control and Prevention)

On-line activities to help young adolescent girls learn about eating and exercise for strong bones.

Website: *www.cdc.gov/powerfulbones*

Take Charge of Your Health: A Teenager's Guide to Better Health (National Institutes of Health)

Information on making healthy food choices and physical activity for teens.

Website: *www.win.niddk.nih.gov/publications/take_charge.htm*

Vegetarian Nutrition for Teenagers (The Vegetarian Resource Group)

Tips from a nutrition expert on eating healthy as a vegetarian.

Website: *www.vrg.org/nutrition/teennutrition.htm*

Your Energy Wake-Up Call: The Simple Solution to Healthy Eating and Activity for Teens (Public Health Institute of California)

Informational site offering ideas to help teens get physically active, scary food facts, recipe files, and tips for student leaders who are ready to make healthy eating a "way of life" at their schools.

Website: *www.caprojectlean.org*

YourSELF Pages for Middle School Students (U.S. Department of Agriculture)

Nutrition education website developed by middle school students for middle school students.

Website: *www.fns.usda.gov/tn/tnrockyrun/default.htm*

4 Girls Health (National Women's Health Information Center)

A website for girls, with lots of information on body, fitness, nutrition, bullying, and a range of topics of relevance to physical, social, and emotional well-being.

Website: *www.4girls.gov*

Organizations

Academy for Eating Disorders
A transdisciplinary professional organization that works to "promote excellence in research, treatment, and prevention of eating disorders."

Address: 6728 Old McLean Village Drive
               McLean, VA 22101
Phone: 703-556-9222
E-mail: *info@aedweb.org*
Website: *www.aedweb.org*

American Dietetic Association
The nation's largest organization of food and nutrition professionals, which "serves the public by promoting optimal nutrition, health, and well-being."

Address: 120 South Riverside Plaza, Suite 2000
               Chicago, IL 60606-6995
Phone: 800-877-1600
Website: *www.eatright.org*

Anorexia Nervosa and Related Eating Disorders, Inc.
A not-for-profit organization that disseminates information about anorexia nervosa, bulimia nervosa, binge eating disorders, and other less well known food and weight disorders.

E-mail: *jarinor@rio.com*
Website: *www.anred.com*

Asian Nutrition Academy
An organization established by health professionals to equip other practitioners with the tools to be experts in nutrition and weight management.

Address: 15A Gold Swan Commercial Building
               438-444 Hennessy Road
               Causeway Bay, Hong Kong
Phone: +852 3427 9727
E-mail: *info@ananutrition.com*
Website: *www.ananutrition.com*

Association for Dietetics in South Africa
An organization of food and nutrition professionals dedicated to using their expertise to promote the nutritional well-being of South Africans.

Address: National Office Secretary
               P.O. Box 81327
               Parkhurst 2120, South Africa

Phone: +27 (0)11 447-4187
E-mail: *adsa@iaafrica.com*
Website: *www.dietetics.co.za./index.html*

Bodywhys

The Irish National Charity dedicated to providing help, support, and understanding to people with eating disorders, their families, and friends and to promoting awareness and understanding among the wider community.

Address: P.O. Box 105
           Blackrock, County Dublin, Ireland
E-mail: *info@bodywhys.ie*
Website: *www.bodywhys.ie*

Center for Weight and Health at the University of California, Berkeley

The Center works to bring together and promote collaboration between researchers, policy makers, and community-based providers from various disciplines and institutions who are concerned with weight, health, and hunger issues.

Address: 101 Giannini Hall #3100
           Berkeley, CA 94720
Phone: 510-642-1599
E-mail: *gwlopez@nature.berkeley.edu*
Website: *nature.berkeley.edu/cwh*

Dads and Daughters

A national nonprofit advocacy organization for fathers and daughters that works to inspire and engage fathers in transforming cultural messages that devalue women.

Address: 34 East Superior Street, Suite 200
           Duluth, MN 55802
Phone: 1-888-824-DADS
E-mail: *Info@dadsanddaughters.org*
Website: *www.dadsanddaughters.org*

Dietitians Association of Australia

DAA is an organization of food and nutrition professionals. The organization's website features information on smart eating, resources for nutrition education, an interactive healthy eating assessment, and links and tools for finding professional services.

Address: 1/8 Phipps Close
           Deuking, ACT 2600, Australia
Phone: 61-2-628 29555
E-mail: *nationaloffice@daa.asn.au*
Website: *www.daa.asn.au*

Eating Disorder Education Organization

A not-for-profit human rights organization working to "increase the awareness of eating disorders and their prevalence throughout society" through education, research, advocacy, computer technology, and member support.

Address: 6R-20 Edmonton General Continuing Care Centre
11111 Jasper Avenue
Edmonton, Alberta T5K 0L4, Canada
Phone: 780-944-2864
E-mail: *infor@edeo.org*
Website: *www.edeo.org*

Eating Disorders Association

A not-for-profit organization that offers information and help for all aspects of eating disorders, including anorexia nervosa, bulimia nervosa, binge eating disorder, and related eating disorders.

Address: 103 Prince of Wales Road
Norwich, Norfolk NR1 1DW, United Kingdom
Phone: +44 1603 619 090
E-mail: *info@edauk.com*
Website: *www.edauk.com*

Eating Disorders Association, Inc. (Queensland)

A nonprofit organization working to improve the intervention, education, and support for all people affected by eating disorders, to raise community awareness about the prevalence and seriousness of these disorders, and to work toward the prevention of eating disorders in our society.

Address: 53 Railway Tce
Milton, Queensland 4064, Australia
Phone: (07) 3876 2500
E-mail: *eda.inc@uq.net.au*
Website: *www.uq.net.au/eda/documents/start.html*

Eating Disorders Association of Manitoba

A nonprofit organization founded to provide support for families and friends of people suffering from eating disorders.

Address: P.O. Box 34099, RPO Fort Richmond
Winnipeg, Manitoba R3T 5T5, Canada
Phone: 204-888-EDAM
Website: *www.edam.mb.ca*

Eating Disorders Wellington

A community-based, not-for-profit organization that serves persons affected by eating disorders, as well as schools, universities, and health professionals, by offering information and resources.

Address: P.O. Box 13 807
           Johnsonville, Wellington, New Zealand
Phone: 04 478 6674
E-mail: *info@eatingdisorders.org.nz*
Website: *www.eatingdisorders.org.nz*

National Eating Disorder Information Centre

A not-for-profit organization that provides information and resources on eating disorders and weight preoccupation

Address: CW 1-211, 200 Elizabeth Street
           Toronto M5G 2C4, Canada
Phone: 1-866-NEDIC-20 (1-866-63342-20)
E-mail: *nedic@uhn.on.ca*
Website: *www.nedic.ca*

National Eating Disorders Association

A not-for-profit organization "working to prevent eating disorders and provide treatment referrals to those suffering from anorexia, bulimia, and binge eating disorder and those concerned with body image and weight issues."

Address: 603 Stewart Street, Suite 803
           Seattle, WA 98101
Phone: 206-382-3587
E-mail: *info@NationalEatingDisorders.org*
Website: *www.nationaleatingdisorders.org*

National Alliance for the Mentally Ill

A not-for-profit, grassroots organization dedicated to the eradication of mental illnesses and enhancing the quality of life for those affected. The organization provides information on eating disorders, related mental illnesses, and psychosocial therapies.

Address: Colonial Place Three
           2107 Wilson Boulevard, Suite 300
           Arlington, VA 22201-3042
Phone: 1-800-950-6264
Website: *www.nami.org*

New Zealand Dietetic Association

An organization of professionals working to promote good health through appropriate food and nutrition.

Address: P.O. Box 5065
            Wellington, New Zealand
Phone: (04) 473 3061
E-mail: *nzda@dietitians.org.nz*
Website: *www.dietitians.org.nz*

Weight Wise (British Dietetic Association)

The British Dietetic Association supports food and nutrition professionals of the United Kingdom and aims to inform the public about nutrition. Weight Wise was designed by these nutrition professionals to give consumers impartial and practical advice and information on managing their weight.

Address: 5th Floor, Charles House
            148/9 Great Charles Street Queensway
            Birmingham B3 3HT, United Kingdom
Phone: 0121 200 8080
E-mail: *info@bda.uk.com*
Websites: *www.bdaweightwise.com*
            www.bda.uk.com/index.html

Women's Sports Foundation

A not-for-profit educational organization dedicated to "ensuring equal access to participation and leadership opportunities for all girls and women in sports and fitness."

Address: Eisenhower Park
            East Meadow, NY 11554
Phone: 1-800-227-3988
E-mail: *wosport@aol.com*
Website: *www.womenssportsfoundation.org*

Bibliography

Chapter 1

Ackard DM, Neumark-Sztainer D, Story M, Perry C. Overeating among adolescents: Prevalence and associations with weight-related characteristics and psychological health. *Pediatrics*. 2003; **111:** 67–74.

American Psychiatric Association. *Diagnostic and statistical manual of mental disorders*, 4th edition (DSM-IV). American Psychiatric Press. Washington, DC. 1994.

Centers for Disease Control. *www.cdc.gov/nccdphp/dash/physicalactivity/guidelines/factsheet.htm*. 2003.

Fairburn CG, Doll HA, Welch SL, Hay PJ, Davies BA, O'Connor ME. Risk factors for binge eating disorder: A community-based case–control study. *Archives of General Psychiatry*. 1998; **55:** 425–432.

Fairburn CG, Welch SL, Doll HA, Davies BA, O'Connor ME. Risk factors for bulimia nervosa: A community-based case–control study. *Archives of General Psychiatry*. 1997; **54:** 509–517.

Field AE, Austin SB, Taylor CB, Malspeis S, Rosner B, Rockett HR, Gillman MW, Colditz, GA. Relation between dieting and weight change among preadolescents and adolescents. *Pediatrics*. 2003; **112**(4): 900–906.

Irving L, Neumark-Sztainer D. Integrating the primary prevention of eating disorders and obesity: Feasible or futile? *Preventive Medicine*. 2002; **34:** 299–309.

Lucas AR, Beard CM, O'Fallon WM, Kurland LT. 50-year trends in the incidence of anorexia nervosa in Rochester, Minnesota: A population-based study. *American Journal of Psychiatry*. 1991; **148:** 917–922.

Michel DM, Willard S. *When dieting becomes dangerous*. Yale University Press. New Haven and London. 2003.

Neumark-Sztainer D. Obesity and eating disorder prevention: An integrated approach? *Adolescent Medicine: State of the Art Reviews (AM:STARS).* 2003; **14:** 159–173.

Neumark-Sztainer D, Story M, Faibisch L, Ohlsen J, Adamiak M. Issues of self-image among overweight African American and Caucasian adolescent girls: A qualitative study. *Journal of Nutrition Education.* 1999; **31**(6): 311–320.

Neumark-Sztainer D, Story M, Hannan PJ, Perry CL, Irving LM. Weight-related concerns and behaviors among overweight and non-overweight adolescents: Implications for preventing weight-related disorders. *Archives of Pediatrics and Adolescent Medicine.* 2002; **156:** 171–178.

Neumark-Sztainer D, Wall M, Story M, Perry C. Correlates of unhealthy weight control behaviors among adolescent girls and boys: Implications for prevention programs. *Health Psychology.* 2003; **22**(1): 88–98.

Nylander I. The feeling of being fat and dieting in a school population: An epidemiological investigation. *Acta Socio-Medica Scandinavica.* . 1971; **1:** 17–26.

Ogden CL, Flegal KM, Carroll MD, Johnson CL. Prevalence and trends in overweight among U.S. children and adolescents, 1999–2000. *Journal of the American Medical Association.* 2002; **288:** 1728–1732.

Ricciardelli LA, McCabe MP. A biopsychosocial model of disordered eating and the pursuit of muscularity in adolescent boys. *Psychological Bulletin.* 2004; **130**(2): 179–205.

Spitzer R, Yanovski S, Wadden T, Wing R, Marcus M, Stunkard A, Devlin M, Hasin D, Horne RL. Binge eating disorder: Its further validation in a multisite study. *International Journal of Eating Disorders,* 1993; **13:** 137–153.

Stein DM. The prevalence of bulimia: A review of the empirical research. *Journal of Nutrition Education.* 1991; **23:** 205–213.

Stice E, Hayward C, Cameron RP, Killen JD, Taylor CB. Body image and eating disturbances predict onset of depression in female adolescents: A longitudinal study. *Journal of Abnormal Psychology.* 2000; **109:** 438–444.

Chapter 2

Ackard DM, Neumark-Sztainer D, Hannan PJ, French S, Story M. Binge and purge behavior among adolescents: Associations with sexual and physical abuse in a nationally representative sample: The Commonwealth Fund survey. *Child Abuse and Neglect.* 2001; **6:** 771–785.

Baumrind, D. The influence of parenting style on adolescent competence and substance use. *Journal of Early Adolescence.* 1991; **11**(1): 56–95.

Birch LL, Davison KK. Family environmental factors influencing the developing behavioral controls of food intake and childhood overweight. *Pediatrics Clinics of North America.* 2001; **48**(4): 893–907.

Birch LL, Fisher JO. Development of eating behaviors among children and adolescents. *Pediatrics.* 1998; **101:** 539–549.

Brewer EA, Kolotkin R, Baird DD. The relationship between eating behaviors and obesity in African American and Caucasian women. *Eating Behaviors*. 2003; **4**: 159–171.

Bronfenbrenner U. Ecology of the family as a context for human development: Research perspectives. *Developmental Psychology*. 1986; **22**: 723–742.

Brownell KD. Dieting and the search for the perfect body: Where physiology and culture collide. *Behavior Therapy*. 1991; **22**: 1–12.

Davison KK, Birch LL. Childhood overweight: A contextual model and recommendations for future research. *Obesity Reviews*. 2001; **2**: 159–171.

Golan M, Crow S. Parents are key players in the prevention and treatment of weight-related problems. *Nutrition Reviews*. 2004; **62**(1): 39–50.

Halmi KA, Sunday SR, Strober M, Kaplan A, Woodside DB, Fichter M, Treasure J, Berrettini WH, Kay WH. Perfectionism in anorexia nervosa: Variation by clinical subtype, obsessionality, and pathological eating behavior. *American Journal of Psychiatry*. 2000; **157**: 1799–1805.

Kelly AM, Wall M, Eisenberg M, Story M, Neumark-Sztainer D. High body satisfaction in adolescent girls: Associations with demographic, socio-environmental, personal and behavioral factors. *Journal of Adolescent Health*. 2004; **34**: 129.

Mellin AE, Neumark-Sztainer D, Patterson J, Sockalosky, J. Unhealthy weight management behaviors among adolescent girls with Type 1 diabetes mellitus: The role of familial eating patterns and weight-related concerns. *Journal of Adolescent Health*. 2004; **35**: 278–289.

Neumark-Sztainer D. Risk factors for childhood and adolescent obesity. *Healthy Generations*. 2000; **1**(2): 3–6.

Neumark-Sztainer D, Story M, Coller T. Perceptions of secondary school staff toward the implementation of school-based activities to prevent weight-related disorders: A needs assessment. *American Journal of Health Promotion*. 1999; **13**(3): 153–156.

Neumark-Sztainer D, Story M, Hannan PJ, Rex J. New Moves: A school-based obesity prevention program for adolescent girls. *Preventive Medicine*. 2003; **37**: 41–51.

Paxton SJ, Schutz HK, Wertheim EH, and Muir SL, Friendship clique and peer influences on body image concerns, dietary restraint, extreme weight loss behaviors, and binge eating in adolescent girls. *Journal of Abnormal Psychology*. 1999; **108**(2): 225–266.

Smolak L, Levine MP. Adolescent transitions and the development of eating problems. In Smolak L, Levine MP, Striegel-Moore R (Eds.). *The developmental psychopathology of eating disorders: Implications for research, prevention, and treatment*. Lawrence Erlbaum Associates, Publishers. Mahwah, NJ. 1996. pp. 207–233.

Striegel-Moore RH, Cachelin FM. Body image concerns and disordered eating in adolescent girls: Risk and protective factors. In Johnson NG, Roberts MC, Worell J (Eds.). *Beyond appearance: A new look at adolescent girls*. American Psychological Association. Washington, DC. 1999. pp. 85–108.

Strober M, Freeman R, Lampert C, Diamond J, Kaye, W. Controlled family study of anorexia nervosa and bulimia nervosa: Evidence of shared liability and transmission of partial syndromes. *American Journal of Psychiatry.* 2000; **157**: 393–401.

Whitaker RC, Wright JA, Pepe MS, Seidel KD, Dietz WH. Predicting obesity in young adulthood from childhood and parental obesity. *New England Journal of Medicine.* 1997; **337**: 869–873.

Chapter 3

Benedikt R, Wertheim E, Love A. Eating attitudes and weight-loss attempts in female adolescents and their mothers. *Journal of Youth and Adolescence.* 1998; **27**(1): 43–57.

Fulkerson JA, McGuire MT, Neumark-Sztainer D, Story M, French SA, Perry CL. Weight-related attitudes and behaviors of adolescent boys and girls who are encouraged to diet by their mothers. *International Journal of Obesity.* 2002; **26**: 1579–1587.

Hanson NI, Neumark-Sztainer D, Eisenberg ME, Story M, Wall M. Associations between parental report of the home food environment and adolescent intakes of fruits, vegetables, and dairy foods. *Public Health Nutrition.* 2005; **8**: 77–85.

Neumark-Sztainer D, Story M, Hannan P, Tharp T, Rex J. Factors associated with changes in physical activity: A cohort study of inactive adolescent girls. *Archives of Pediatrics and Adolescent Medicine.* 2003; **157**: 803–810.

Neumark-Sztainer D, Wall M, Story M, Perry CL. Correlates of unhealthy weight-control behaviors among adolescents: Implications for prevention programs. *Health Psychology.* 2003; **22**(1): 88–98.

Paikoff R, Brooks-Gunn J, Carlton-Ford S. Effect of reproductive status changes upon family functioning and well-being of mothers and daughters. *Journal of Early Adolescence.* 1991; **11**: 201–220.

Sallis JF, Prochaska JJ, Taylor WC. A review of correlates of physical activity of children and adolescents. *Medicine and Science in Sports and Exercise.* 2000; **32**: 963–975.

Wertheim EH, Martin G, Prior M, Sanson A, Smart D. Parent influences in the transmission of eating and weight-related values and behaviors. *Eating Disorders: The Journal of Treatment and Prevention.* 2002; **10**: 321–324.

Wertheim EH, Mee V, Paxton SJ. Relationships among adolescent girls' eating behaviors and their parents' weight-related attitudes and behaviors. *Sex Roles.* 1999; **41**: 169–187.

Chapter 4

Andersen, AE, DiDomenico, L. Diet vs. shape content of popular male and female magazines: A dose–response relationship to the incidence of eating disorders? *International Journal of Eating Disorders.* 1992; **11**(3): 283–287.

Becker AE, Burwell RA, Gilman SE, Herzog DB, Hamburg P. Eating behaviours and attitudes following prolonged exposure to television among ethnic Fijian adolescent girls. *British Journal of Psychiatry.* 2002; **180:** 509–514.

Braun DL, Sunday SR, Huang A, Halmi KA. More males seek treatment for eating disorders. *International Journal of Eating Disorders.* 1999; **25:** 415–424.

Dennison BA, Erb TA, Jenkins PL. Television viewing and television in bedroom associated with overweight risk among low-income preschool children. *Pediatrics.* 2002: **109**(6): 1028–1035.

Eisenberg M, Neumark-Sztainer D, Story M. Associations of weight-based teasing and emotional well-being among adolescents. *Archives of Pediatrics and Adolescent Medicine.* 2003; **157:** 733–738.

Friedman SS. *When girls feel fat: Helping girls through adolescence.* HarperCollins. Toronto. 1997.

Neumark-Sztainer D, Falkner N, Story M, Perry C, Hannan P, Mulert S. Weight-teasing among adolescents: Correlations with weight status and disordered eating behaviors. *International Journal of Obesity.* 2002; **26**(1): 123–131.

Neumark-Sztainer D, Sherwood N, Coller T, Hannan P. Primary prevention of disordered eating among pre-adolescent girls: Feasibility and short-term impact of a community-based intervention. *Journal of the American Dietetic Association.* 2000; **100**(12): 1466–1473.

Neumark-Sztainer D, Story M, Faibisch L, Ohlson J, Adamiak M. Issues of self-image among overweight African American and Caucasian girls: A qualitative study. *Journal of Nutrition Education.* 1999; **31:** 311–320.

Neumark-Sztainer D, Story M, Faibisch L. Perceived stigmatization among overweight African-American and Caucasian adolescent girls. *Journal of Adolescent Health.* 1998; **23:** 264–270.

Paxton SJ, Schutz HK, Wertheim EH, Muir SL. Friendship clique and peer influences on body image concerns. Dietary restraint, extreme weight loss behaviors, and binge eating in adolescent girls. *Journal of Abnormal Psychology.* 1999; **108**(2): 255–266.

Pope HG, Olivardia R, Gruber A, Borowiecki J. Evolving ideals of male body image as seen through action toys. *International Journal of Eating Disorders.* 1999; **26:** 65–72.

Saelens BE, Sallis JF, Nader PR, Broyles SL, Berry CC, Taras HL. Home and environmental influences on children's television watching from early to middle childhood. *Journal of Developmental and Behavioral Pediatrics.* 2002; **23**(3): 127–132.

Schlenker J, Caron SL, Halteman WA. A feminist analysis of *Seventeen* magazine: Content analysis from 1945 to 1995. *Sex Roles.* 1998; **38:** 135–149.

Utter J, Neumark-Sztainer D, Wall M, Story M. Reading magazine articles about dieting and associated weight control behaviors among adolescents. *Journal of Adolescent Health.* 2003; **32:** 78–82.

Wertheim EH, Paxton SJ, Schutz HK, Muir SL. Why do adolescent girls watch their weight? An interview study examining sociocultural pressures to be thin. *Journal of Psychosomatic Research*. 1997; **42**(4): 345–355.

Wiecha JL, Sobol AM, Peterson KE, Gortmaker SL. Household television access: Associations with screen time, reading, and homework among youth. *Ambulatory Pediatrics*. 2001; **1**(5): 244–251.

Chapter 5

Centers for Disease Control. *www.cdc.gov/nccdphp/dash/physicalactivity/guidelines/factsheet.htm*. 2003.

Centers for Disease Control. *www.cdc.gov/nccdphp/dash/physicalactivity/promoting_health/background.htm*. 2003.

Centers for Disease Control and Prevention. *Surveillance Summaries*, June 28, 2002. MMWR 2002: 51(No. SS-4).

Faith MS, Leone MA, Ayers TS, Heo M, Pietrobelli A. Weight criticism during physical activity, coping skills, and reported physical activity in children. *Pediatrics* 2002; **110**(2): 23.

Johnston LD, O'Malley PM, Bachman, JG. (2003). *Monitoring the Future national results on adolescent drug use: Overview of key findings, 2002* (NIH Publication No. 03–5374). National Institute on Drug Abuse. Bethesda, MD.

Kaiser Family Foundation. *Kids & media @ the new millenium* [monograph]. Kaiser Family Foundation. Menlo Park, CA. November 1999.

Kimm SYS, Glynn NW, Kriska AM, Barton BA, Kronsberg SS, Daniels SR, Crawford PB, Sabry ZI, Liu K. Decline in physical activity in black girls and white girls during adolescence. *New England Journal of Medicine*. 2002; **347**: 709–715.

Irving LM, Wall M, Neumark-Sztainer D, Story M. Steroid use among adolescents: Findings from Project EAT. *Journal of Adolescent Health*. 2002; **30**: 243–252.

Neumark-Sztainer D, Story M, Hannan PJ, Rex J. New Moves: A school-based obesity prevention program for adolescent girls. *Preventive Medicine*. 2003; **37**: 41–51.

Ogden CL, Flegal KM, Carroll MD, Johnson CL. Prevalence and trends in overweight among U.S. children and adolescents, 1999–2000. *Journal of the American Medical Association*. 2002; **288**: 1728–1732.

Powers PS. Athletes and eating disorders. *Eating Disorders: The Journal of Treatment and Prevention*. 1999; **7**: 249–255.

Sallis JF, Patrick K. Physical activity guidelines for adolescents: Consensus statement. *Pediatric Exercise Science*. 1994; **6**: 302–314.

Sherwood N, Neumark-Sztainer D, Story M, Beuhring T, Resnick M. Weight-related sports involvement in girls: Who is at risk for disordered eating? *American Journal of Health Promotion*. 2002; **16**(6): 341–344.

Smolak L, Murnen SK, Ruble AE. Female athletes and eating problems: A meta-analysis. *International Journal of Eating Disorders*. 2000; **27**: 371–380.

Story M, Holt K, Sofka D. (Eds.). *Bright futures in practice: Nutrition*, 2nd edition. National Center for Education in Maternal and Child Health. Arlington, VA. 2002.

Taylor WC, Yancey AK, Leslie J, Murray NG, Cummings SS, Sharkey SA, Wert C, James J, Miles O, McCarthy WJ. Physical activity among African American and Latino middle school girls: Consistent beliefs, expectations, and experiences across two sites. *Women Health*. 1999; **30**: 67–82.

Thompson RA, Sherman RT. "Good athlete" traits and characteristics of anorexia nervosa: Are they similar? *Eating Disorders*.1999: **7**: 181–190.

Tiggemann M. The impact of adolescent girls' life concerns and leisure activities on body dissatisfaction, disordered eating, and self-esteem. *Journal of Genetic Psychology*. 2001; **162**(2): 133–142.

U.S. Department of Agriculture and U.S. Department of Health and Human Services. *Nutrition and your health: Dietary guidelines for Americans* (5th ed.). U.S. Department of Agriculture and U.S. Department of Health and Human Services, U.S. Government Printing Office. Washington, DC. 2000.

U.S. Department of Health and Human Services. *Anabolic steroid abuse*. National Institutes of Health. Washington, DC. 2000.

U.S. Department of Transportation, Federal Highway Administration, Research and Technical Support Center. *Nationwide Personal Transportation Survey*. Federal Highway Administration. Lantham, MD 1997.

Chapter 6

Field AE, Austin SB, Taylor CB, Malspeis S, Rosner B, Rockett HR, Gillman MW, Colditz, GA. Relation between dieting and weight change among preadolescents and adolescents. *Pediatrics*. 2003; **112**(4): 900–906.

Kadlec D. The low-carb frenzy. *Time*. 2004; **163**(18): 46–54.

Neumark-Sztainer D, Bulter R, Palti H. Dieting and binge-eating: Which dieters are at risk? *Journal of the American Dietetic Association*. 1995; **95**(5): 586–589.

Neumark-Sztainer D, Hannan P. Weight-related behaviors among adolescent girls and boys. *Archives of Pediatrics and Adolescent Medicine*. 2000; **154**: 569–577.

Neumark-Sztainer D, Hannan P, Story M, Perry C. Weight control behaviors among adolescent girls and boys: Implications for dietary intake. *Journal of the American Dietetic Association*. 2004; **104**: 913–920.

Neumark-Sztainer D, Story M. Dieting and binge eating among adolescents: What do they really mean? *Journal of the American Dietetic Association*. 1998; **98**: 446–450.

Nichter M. *Fat talk*. Harvard University Press. Cambridge, MA. 2000.

Nylander I. The feeling of being fat and dieting in a school population: An epidemiologic interview investigation. *Acta Socio-Medica Scandinavica*. 1971; **1**: 17–26.

Patton GC, Seizer R, Coffey C, Carlin JB, Wolfe R. Onset of adolescent eating disorders: population based cohort study over 3 years. *British Medical Journal*. 1999; **318**: 765–768.

Stice E, Cameron RP, Killen JD, Hayward C, Taylor CB. Naturalistic weight-reduction efforts prospectively predict growth in relative weight and onset of obesity among female adolescents. *Journal of Consulting and Clinical Psychology*. 1999; **67**(6): 967–974.

Stice E, Hayward C, Cameron R, Killen JD, Taylor CB. Body image and eating disturbances predict onset of depression in female adolescents: A longitudinal study.
Journal of Abnormal Psychology. 2000; **109:** 438–444.

Wing RR, Hill JO. Successful weight loss maintenance. *Annual Reviews of Nutrition.*
2001; **21:** 323–341.

Chapter 8

Birch LL, Fisher JO, Davison KK. Learning to overeat: Maternal use of restrictive
feeding practices promotes girls' eating in the absence of hunger. *American Journal of Clinical Nutrition.* 2003; **78**(2): 215–220.

Hanson NI, Neumark-Sztainer D, Eisenberg ME, Story M, Wall M. Associations between parental report of the home food environment and adolescent intakes of
fruits, vegetables, and dairy foods. *Public Health Nutrition.* 2005; **8:** 77-85.

Munoz KA, Krebs-Smith SM, Ballard-Barbash R, Cleveland LE. Food intakes of US
children and adolescents compared with recommendations [published erratum
appears in *Pediatrics.* 1998; **101:** 952–953]. *Pediatrics.* 1997; 100: 323–329.

Neumark-Sztainer D, Story M, Hannan PJ, Croll J. Overweight status and eating patterns among adolescents: Where do youths stand in comparison with the Healthy
People 2010 Objectives? *American Journal of Public Health.* 2002; **92:** 844–851.

Neumark-Sztainer D, Wall M, Perry C, Story M. Correlates of fruit and vegetable intake among adolescents: Findings from Project EAT. *Preventive Medicine.* 2003;
37: 198–208.

Story M. Nutritional requirements during adolescence. In McAnarney ER, Kreipe RE,
Orr DE, Comerci DG (Eds.). *Textbook of adolescent medicine.* WB Saunders. Philadelphia. 1992. pp. 75–84.

Story M, Holt K, Sofka D. (Eds.). *Bright futures in practice: Nutrition,* 2nd edition. National Center for Education in Maternal and Child Health. Arlington, VA. 2002.

Story M, Resnick MD. Adolescents' views on food and nutrition. *Journal of Nutrition
Education.* 1986; **18**(4): 188–192.

U.S. Department of Agriculture. *Food and nutrient intakes by children 1994–96, 1998.*
ARS Food Surveys Research Group. Beltsville, MD. 1999.

U.S. Department of Agriculture and U.S. Department of Health and Human Services.
Nutrition and your health: Dietary guidelines for Americans (5th ed.). U.S. Department of Agriculture and U.S. Department of Health and Human Services. Washington, DC. 2000.

Chapter 9

Satter E. *How to get your kid to eat . . . but not too much.* Bull Publishing. Boulder, CO.
1987.

Nielsen SJ, Popkin BM. Patterns and trends in food portion sizes, 1977–1998. *Journal
of the American Medical Association.* 2003; **289:** 450–453.

Rolls BJ. The supersizing of America: Portion size and the obesity epidemic. *Nutrition Today.* 2003; **38**(2): 42–52.

Rolls BJ, Morris El, Roe, LA. Portion size of food affects energy intake in normal-weight and overweight men and women. *American Journal of Clinical Nutrition.* 2002; **76:** 1207–1213.

Rolls LL, Engell D, Birch LL. Serving portion size influences 5–year old but not 3-year-old children's food intakes. *Journal of the American Dietetic Association.* 2000; **100:** 232–234.

Young LR, Nestle M. The contribution of expanding portion sizes to the U.S. obesity epidemic. *American Journal of Public Health.* 2002; **92**(2): 246–249.

Chapter 10

Klopp SA, Heiss CJ, Smith HS. Self-reported vegetarianism may be a marker for college women at risk for disordered eating. *Journal of the American Dietetic Association.* 2003; **103:** 745–747.

Lappe FM. *Diet for a small planet.* Ballantine Books. New York. 1991.

Mangels AR, Messina V, Melina V. Position of the American Dietetic Association and Dietitians of Canada: Vegetarian diets. *Journal of the American Dietetic Association.* 2003; **103**(6): 748–765.

Messina V, Melina V, Mangels AR. A new food guide for North American vegetarians. *Journal of the American Dietetic Association.* 2003; **103**(6): 771–775.

Messina VK, Burke KI. Position of the American Dietetic Association: Vegetarian diets. *Journal of the American Dietetic Association.* 1997; **97**(11): 1317–1321.

Neumark-Sztainer D, Story M, Resnick MD, Blum RW. Adolescent vegetarians: A behavioral profile of a school-based population in Minnesota. *Archives of Pediatrics and Adolescent Medicine.* 1997; **151:** 833–838.

O'Connor MA, Touyz SW, Dunn SM, Beumont PJV. Vegetarianism in anorexia nervosa? A review of 116 consecutive cases. *Medical Journal of Australia.* 1987; **147:** 540–542.

Perry CL, Lytle LA, Jacobs T. *The vegetarian manifesto.* Running Press. Philadephia. 2004.

Perry CL, McGuire MT, Neumark-Sztainer D, Story M. Characteristics of vegetarian adolescents in a multiethnic urban population. *Journal of Adolescent Health.* 2001; **29:** 406–416.

Perry CL, McGuire MT, Neumark-Sztainer D, Story M. Adolescent vegetarians: How well do their dietary patterns meet the Healthy People 2010 objectives? *Archives of Pediatrics and Adolescent Medicine.* 2002; 156: 431–437.

Chapter 11

Ackard DM, Neumark-Sztainer D. Family mealtime while growing up: Associations with symptoms of bulimia nervosa. *Eating Disorders.* 2001; **9:** 239–249.

Eisenberg ME, Olson RE, Neumark-Sztainer D, Story M, Bearinger L. Correlations between family meals and psychosocial well-being among adolescents. *Archives of Pediatrics and Adolescent Medicine.* 2004; **158**: 792–796.

Gillman MW, Rifas-Shiman SL, Frazier L, Rockett HRH, Camargo CA, Field AE, Berkey CS, Colditz GA. Family dinner and diet quality among older children and adolescents. *Archives of Family Medicine.* 2000; 9: 235–240.

Neumark-Sztainer D, Hannan PJ, Story M, Croll J, Perry C. Family meal patterns: Associations with sociodemographic characteristics and improved dietary intake among adolescents. *Journal of the American Dietetic Association.* 2003; **3**: 317–322.

Neumark-Sztainer D, Story M, Ackard D, Moe J, Perry C. The "family meal": Views of adolescents. *Journal of Nutrition Education.* 2000a; **32**: 329–334.

Neumark-Sztainer D, Story M, Ackard D, Moe J, Perry C. Family meals among adolescents: Findings from a pilot study. *Journal of Nutrition Education.* 2000b; **32**: 355–340.

Neumark-Sztainer D, Wall M, Story M, Fulkerson J. Are family meal patterns associated with disordered eating behaviors among adolescents? *Journal of Adolescent Health.* 2004; **35**: 350–359.

Chapter 12

Bowman SA, Gortmaker SL, Ebbeling CB, Pereira MA, Ludwig DS. Effects of fast-food consumption on energy intake and diet quality among children in a national household survey. *Pediatrics.* 2004; **113**: 112–118.

French SA, Story M, Neumark-Sztainer D, Fulkerson JA, Hannan P. Fast food restaurant use among adolescents: Associations with nutrient intake, food choices, behavioral and psychosocial variables. *International Journal of Obesity* 2001; **25**: 1823–2833.

Jacobson MF, Hurley JG, and the Center for Science in the Public Interest. *Restaurant confidential.* Workman Publishing. New York. 2002.

Lin BH, Guthrie JF, Blaylock J. *The diets of America's children: Influences of dining out, household characteristics, and nutrition knowledge* (U.S. Department of Agriculture, Economic Report No. 746 [AER-746]). U.S. Department of Agriculture. Washington, DC. 1996.

Lin BH, Guthrie JF, Frazao E. Nutrient contribution of food away from home. In Frazao E (Ed.). *America's eating habits: Changes and consequences.* U.S. Department of Agriculture. Washington, DC. 1999. pp. 213–242.

Lin BH, Guthrie JF, Frazao E. Quality of children's diets at and away from home: 1994–96. *Food Review.* 1999; **22**(1): 2–10.

National Restaurant Association. *Restaurant industry pocket fact-book. www.restaurant.org/store/C1660.html.* 2000.

National Restaurant Association. *2004 Restaurant industry forecast.* Executive summary. *www.restaurant.org/pdfs/research/2004_forecast_execsummary.pdf.* 2004.

Chapter 13

Ackard DM, Neumark-Sztainer D. Health care information sources for adolescents: Age and gender differences on use, concerns, and needs. *Journal of Adolescent Health*. 2001; **29**(3): 170–176.

Neumark-Sztainer D, Story M, Hannan PJ, Beuhring T, Resnick MD. Disordered eating among adolescents: Associations with sexual/physical abuse and other familial/psychosocial factors. *International Journal of Eating Disorders*. 2000; **20**: 249–258.

Chapter 14

Mellin A, Neumark-Sztainer D, Story M, Ireland M, Resnick M. Unhealthy behaviors and psychosocial difficulties among overweight youth: The potential impact of familial factors. *Journal of Adolescent Health*. 2002; **31**: 145–153.

Neumark-Sztainer D, Goeden C, Story M, Wall M. Associations between body satisfaction and physical activity in adolescents: Implications for programs aimed at preventing a broad spectrum of weight-related disorders. *Eating Disorders: The Journal of Treatment and Prevention*. 2004; **12**: 125–137.

Neumark-Sztainer D, Martin SL, Story M. School-based programs for obesity prevention: What do adolescents recommend? *American Journal of Health Promotion*. 2000; **14**(4): 232–235.

Neumark-Sztainer D, Story M. Recommendations from overweight youth regarding school-based weight control programs. *Journal of School Health*. 1997; **67**(10): 428–433.

Neumark-Sztainer D, Story M, Faibisch L. Perceived stigmatization among overweight African-American and Caucasian adolescent girls. *Journal of Adolescent Health*. 1998; **23**: 264–270.

Neumark-Sztainer D, Story M, Faibisch L, Ohlsen J, Adamiak M. Issues of self-image among overweight African American and Caucasian adolescent girls: A qualitative study. *Journal of Nutrition Education*. 1999; **31**(6): 311–320.

Neumark-Sztainer D, Story M, Hannan PJ, Rex J. New Moves: A school-based obesity prevention program for adolescent girls. *Preventive Medicine*. 2003; **37**: 41–51.

Sobal J. Obesity and nutritional sociology: A model for coping with the stigma of obesity. *Clinical Sociology Review*. 1991; **9**: 125–141.

Chapter 15

Ackard DM, Neumark-Sztainer D. Multiple sexual victimizations among adolescent boys and girls: Prevalence and associations with eating behaviors and psychological health. *Journal of Child Sexual Abuse*. 2003: **12**(1): 17–37.

French SA, Story M, Remafedi G, Resnick MD, Blum RW. Sexual orientation and

Bibliography

prevalence of body dissatisfaction and eating disordered behaviors: A population-based study of adolescents. *International Journal of Eating Disorders*. 1996; **19**(2): 119–126.

Mellin AE, Neumark-Sztainer D, Patterson J. Parenting adolescent girls with Type 1 diabetes: Parents' perspectives. *Journal of Pediatric Psychology*. 2004; **29**(3): 221–230.

Mellin AE, Neumark-Sztainer D, Patterson J, Sockalosky, J. Unhealthy weight management behaviors among adolescent girls with Type 1 diabetes mellitus: The role of familial eating patterns and weight-related concerns. *Journal of Adolescent Health*. 2004; **35**: 278–289.

Neumark-Sztainer D, Patterson J, Mellin A, Ackard DM, Utter J, Story M, Sockalosky J. Weight control practices and disordered eating behaviors among adolescent females and males with Type 1 diabetes: Associations with sociodemographics, weight concerns, familial factors, and metabolic outcomes. *Diabetes Care*. 2002; **5**(8): 1289–1296.

Neumark-Sztainer D, Story M, Garwick A, Resnick MD, Blum RW. Body dissatisfaction and unhealthy weight control practices among adolescents with and without chronic illness: A population-based study. *Archives of Pediatrics and Adolescent Medicine*. 1995; **149**: 1330–1335.

Rob AS, Dadson MJ. Eating disorders in males. *Child and Adolescent Psychiatric Clinics of North America*. 2002; **11**(2): 399–418.

Rodin G, Olmsted MP, Rydall AC, Maharaj SI, Colton PA, Jones JM, Biancucci LA, Daneman D. Eating disorders in young women with Type 1 diabetes mellitus. *Journal of Psychosomatic Research*. 2002; **53**(4): 943–949.

Russell CJ, Keel PK. Homosexuality as a specific risk factor for eating disorders in men. *International Journal of Eating Disorders*. 2002; **31**(3): 300–306.

Index

Index

313

About the Author

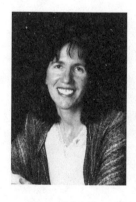

Dianne Neumark-Sztainer, PhD, MPH, RD, is a Professor in the Division of Epidemiology and Community Health, School of Public Health, and an Adjunct Professor in the Department of Pediatrics, School of Medicine, at the University of Minnesota. Her research focuses on eating disorder and obesity prevention in teenagers and on understanding factors associated with eating patterns, physical activity, dieting behaviors, and body image in teens. Dr. Neumark-Sztainer has published some 150 research articles in scientific journals such as the *American Journal of Public Health*, *Health Psychology*, *Preventive Medicine*, *Journal of Adolescent Health*, and *Journal of the American Dietetic Association*. She has authored several curriculum programs aimed at the prevention of different weight-related problems in children and teens for schools and Girl Scout programs. Dr. Neumark-Sztainer has presented her research throughout the United States and in Canada, Australia, Israel, and various European countries. Her work is often featured in newspapers, radio shows, and television programs. She lived in Israel for over a decade and now lives in Minnesota with her husband and their four children, who are at different stages of adolescence.

317